If you want to know more about how to do the work of professional care-giving, to learn more about real-life psychology underpinning effective care-work, and or to further foster your understanding of giving and receiving care as a reflective practitioner, this is a must read text for you. It offers direct access and refreshing insight into the world of mental health drawing upon a wide range of rich experience. It should inspire student, professional or interested reader alike in facilitating further their own development, personal thinking and relevant reflective practice. I suggest this is a book to own, use and re-use as a tool for teaching and a practical source for what is a serial series of learning conversation about the work of mental health and pastoral care.

Professor Emeritus Stephen Rayner,
Birmingham Newman University, UK

There is something profoundly humbling about being called to serve others. Not just as a teacher to teach, or a psychologist to treat (both of which imply a certain status in the relationship) but to share, sit with, support and serve others in their moments of need. Through rich case explorations and thought provoking questions, Dr Esther Roodenburg continues to serve and help other psychologists to serve.

Dr Shane Costello, *Educational and Developmental Psychologist,*
Adjunct Senior Lecturer, Monash University, Australia

A Psychologist's Casebook

Drawing on examples from clinical practice, this book presents evidence-based psychological principles in an applied context to support effective practice in the helping professions.

This book takes a narrative approach, presenting a collection of individual cases to complement the traditionally theory-heavy education and training of mental health professionals. It demonstrates easy to learn, practical skills found invaluable in supporting and treating a broad range of clients, from pre-verbal children to the elderly. The case examples are designed to encourage and motivate a more comprehensive understanding of general psychological terms, which is further supported by callouts, reflection prompts, and extension exercises.

Rich with examples from the authors' many years of clinical psychology practice and graduate teaching, this book is written for students and practitioners alike.

Esther M Roodenburg is a former academic at Monash University, Australia, who remains committed to community involvement. After secondary teaching, and raising five children, she continued her work as a community-based psychologist, completing a qualitative PhD researching individual differences. Her university graduate teaching and supervision focused on broad case-based practical applications of evidence-based therapeutic approaches.

John Roodenburg was awarded the 2020 APS National Award of Distinction for leadership in Educational and Developmental Psychology while an academic and clinic director at Monash University. Primary school teaching was followed by work as a school psychologist in rural Victoria. Graduate-level teaching followed his completion of a PhD modelling individual differences in thinking.

A Psychologist's Casebook

Cases from Practice Used to Support Teaching Mental Health Practitioners

Esther M Roodenburg with
John Roodenburg

Routledge
Taylor & Francis Group
LONDON AND NEW YORK

Designed cover image: Getty

First published 2025
by Routledge
4 Park Square, Milton Park, Abingdon, Oxon OX14 4RN

and by Routledge
605 Third Avenue, New York, NY 10158

Routledge is an imprint of the Taylor & Francis Group, an informa business

British Library Cataloguing-in-Publication Data
A catalogue record for this book is available from the British Library

ISBN: 9781032755564 (hbk)
ISBN: 9781032755540 (pbk)
ISBN: 9781003474746 (ebk)

DOI: 10.4324/9781003474746

Typeset in Times New Roman
by codeMantra

This book is written in service to those many people who gladly give so that others may experience more of a life well lived. It is hoped that each reader will also be encouraged to know more of the Supreme Being who continues to assure us that it is more blessed to give than to receive.

Contents

Foreword

"I have mulled over the idea of my writing a foreword and honestly think it would be a mistake to insert my voice at the front of the book. I think much of the 'power' of the book rests with its 'narrative' style and the clear, direct, and personal nature of your authorial voice. I suggest this would be interrupted inappropriately by another voice with a foreword... I have therefore not written a foreword... BW. Steve."

Professor Emeritus Stephen Rayner,
Birmingham Newman University, UK

Preface

In facing retirement, the desire to continue to be useful hit me: how could I stop being who I am, a person who loves people and loves enabling others to reach their potential, simply because my paid work has ended? Should I now seek to find satisfaction in finding and taking up new tools, such as those needed for gardening? Should I forget about those many tools that have been essential to keep honed when dealing with an incredible variety of people and their individual needs? After all, these tools were developed over many years, first as a *teacher*, then as a *parent* of five quite different and challengingly wonderful children, while I continued as a *practising psychologist* (an interesting descriptor, isn't it – implies keeping it up or losing it!).

While I at the same time completed my own research into individual differences in the ways people think, the last ten-plus years have continued my desire to serve, made possible through the opportunity to share many of those same skills with graduate psychologists in training within a university. This involved teaching both enthusiastic younger learners already in their chosen careers, and many mature-aged psychologists, having returned for further professional development. Almost all of these students we have found to be impressively committed to better understanding of and engagement with their clients.

As the questions concerning post-employment became clearer with time, opportunities also arose for engaging within local communities. But volunteers are often assumed to have few professionally developed skills. In reality, how could my engagement with other volunteers then be constructive within the community, and not in any way be threatening? Alternatively, in addition to the joy of picking up new interests and skills, I was left asking, what should I do with my practice skills – could these still be of use to others?

Ah, yes – another ubiquitous book. Even the writer of Ecclesiastes once said: "of the making of books there will be no end."[1] While teaching I had frequent requests for practical, informative case studies – these were found to be fundamental to providing practical examples that support the theories students had already become saturated with.

So, in setting the stage for what I hope will be a useful collection of my reflections of the insights and skills gained through practice, there are several points that need to be made.

Firstly, "cases" are variously presented, some as composites of counselling experiences, and all are referred to with fictitious names and places. Details that might in any way potentially identify anyone have been carefully and appropriately altered. Any composite cases are made up of truthful accounts of what individual clients shared, with my honest reflections on the success or failure of specific therapeutic approaches used, so that the authenticity of the associated skills required can be assessed by the reader.

It also needs to be said that this book is not about me: it is about the people whose life stories have contributed to the case studies, with samples of what can be done for people seeking help. Each experience has been selected to illustrate issues that at times required quite differing techniques. I make no apology for rarely including personal comments, other than as necessary to explain chosen therapies or reactions drawn from me.

It is also important to note that throughout the book, sometimes cases are referred to as "clients", acknowledging a professional relationship expected of "the helper" with whom the one wanting help has agreed to engage. So with this in mind, you as the helper may need to reflect on your role and your own relationship with those you seek to help.

Another book, yes, but one that hopefully provides some practical insights about potential tools needed, particularly for those would-be people helpers such as young psychologists, chaplains in training, or other health professionals who are keen to learn from others' lived experiences and may be further inspired as they commit to becoming more effective. Many of us learn by reflecting on anecdotes that clearly come from everyday scenarios, and these can both support and humanise the book learning that is often theoretical and somewhat detached. The reader may find that many of these stories may be readily applied to everyday personal life experiences, whether within an urban or rural setting, being as relevant to the poor as to the wealthy, and appropriate for youth and equally to the elderly.

It needs to be acknowledged here that it was never my intention to write yet another textbook. There are already many such valuable resources, some of which will be mentioned should the reader need to investigate the techniques and tools used herein, and from a more theoretical perspective.

It is with this hope in mind that I dare to record and make public some of the amazing things learnt, having been privileged to journey with so many wonderful people who trusted me enough to share their difficulties and many, their subsequent joys. I also hope you will grasp throughout these reflections the importance of maintaining an attitude of care and acceptance, regardless of how one may disagree with others' values and beliefs.

The text is written in the first person, but joining me in this project, adding his experiences and perspectives, is psychologist, colleague, and dear friend, my husband, John. Without his incredible support and his experiences included, this book would never have been written.

Esther M Roodenburg Melbourne,
Australia, June 2024

Note

1 Biblical wise sayings on life's futilities: Ecclesiastes 12: 12.

Chapter 1

Where do we begin?

Setting the stage for reflections on a shared journey with others, this chapter looks at some of the concerns people often have about what may be encountered, and how they may be prepared to deal with these potential hurdles. Not only is the motivation question "why are we taking this pathway" necessary, but it supports our asking what some of the relevant personal probes about the past may reveal, useful for both the helper and those seeking assistance. As a pattern used throughout the book, various clients will be discussed here to encourage the reader in considering how prepared he/she is to handle the challenges, how ready to dig more deeply into any apparent issue presented. A pattern of learning through reflective exercises is adopted in each chapter. This first one asks: how well do we understand that our being successful caregivers rests on our being effective listeners?

Do you ever wonder what motivates many of us who seek to help others? Surely this question is the first port of call as we begin a book of reflections on people encountered on our journey. But wait! Why do we need to reflect? Don't we need to be looking forward, forgetting the things behind and simply press on?

Historians however are the first to tell us that without reflecting on the past we will simply repeat the same mistakes again and again. Think about repeated disasters created by governments, or families that generation after generation seem incapable of turning the tide against bad destructive patterns of behaviour. So, let's consider in what ways the main events of the past may have led us personally on this journey of helping others. We may also like to challenge the oft-quoted belief that 'past behaviour is the best predictor of future behaviour'; otherwise, we might not continue to believe our work makes any difference.

On reflection, we may have experienced support from someone at a particular time that may explain why we aspire to do similarly wonderful things to help others. Almost like giving back because we've been given to. Or perhaps we wish there *had* been support available, when at some point in our history there had been none, so had to struggle on alone. This alternate motivation can also be a good thing, and for some of us has meant that we began the journey to find out

DOI: 10.4324/9781003474746-1

things we would like to have known earlier. We convince ourselves that in trying to understand our own past, we may at the same time help others.

Perhaps we simply like helping people, particularly those who may have been offended or hurt through no fault of their own. After all, our family was always good at doing things for others, and we found that a good model to emulate. Surely this too is a noble motivation, and admittedly one that is commonly felt and acted upon.

> *Reflect now on your own motivation: clarify it, so you don't get caught out by being subconsciously unaware of what really drives you.*

Motivation

As alluded to in the foreword, my personal motivation in writing this book is to share some of the varied examples of the sorts of problems that individuals bring to their psychologist. Many clients bring with them unexplored or unrealistic expectations about what will be achieved, and for their sake as well as mine, these need to be brought out into the open. All examples are based on true stories, shared with me within a rural setting in Australia but given here as vignettes only, to demonstrate anecdotally some of the skills needed if we are to support others. At the same time, these stories are presented as a way of encouraging you the reader to learn to be reflective and adaptable. They will be representative of the many very real people with whom we all cross paths. Given the wide range of individual differences in those we meet (for example in appearance, cultural backgrounds, values, and religious beliefs), our role as people helpers, supporters, and counsellors will always demand a wide set of tools that can be carefully selected as we become increasingly aware of individual orientations and needs.

In this first chapter, I hope to whet your appetite for the later chapters which focus on the more specific ways of utilising the various options that are only briefly mentioned in these initial cases. But even when we become more competent in understanding these various basic tools, I would like to begin with an acknowledgement that as people helpers, we should never expect to have the right answers. It is not about us, nor about the answers we think we may have. To be effective, we accept that we are called to relate to people as individuals, each as uniquely different as the fingerprints which identify them. Though we are also committed to understanding people, it is never to be in judgement. Our commonly expressed human reaction can so easily suggest that certain people should just be pulled into line, since their behaviour is unacceptable, at least to us! But if we hope to reach our clients in the best way possible, being critical will simply confirm what that person has undoubtedly heard from others. It may in fact be why they still struggle, craving a more loving, careful understanding before daring to make changes.

We have our own beliefs and values, and ones we may legitimately consider to give us clear insights into what are destructive and damaging attitudes and behaviours that need attention. But if we are to help others, unconditional acceptance of them as individuals is paramount. This is not to suggest that we are simply to be permissive or undiscerning about difficult behaviours. While appropriately supporting individuals, we may find it appropriate to challenge them with the need to accept personal responsibility for change. But, regardless of how we *feel* towards the individual's behaviour or the values conflict we perceive, a helper's role is never to be the authoritarian, acting as judge and jury. Much is available about this in textbooks on counselling for helping people responsibly to effect positive change.

Depending on your values and beliefs, past experiences that still worry you, or (dare I say it?) a seemingly difficult clash of personalities, someone else might better serve the person you'd like to help. An honest appraisal creates respect, even if one is not liked for it!

I recall one client who had a clear agenda: to engage my support for a compensation claim against an employer. Ray had hated his place of work, and had always intended to retire by age 55, because he wanted to travel. It soon became clear that his way out was to make an exaggerated claim about an injury which he had lived with for many years – a leg injury which meant he preferred to sit, rather than stand, while working. Agreement had been made by his supermarket manager to have that problem removed, arranging a chair at the checkout, but for Ray this wasn't enough. He wanted a monetary compensation, and he needed my cooperation, asking that I make a report to support this demand. A couple of sessions only were needed to determine that this man's motivation was blatantly dishonest, and he may have thought that my being a woman meant he could manipulate me for his own ends. Eventual honesty allowed me to be equally honest: there was no way I could support his claim, so he left, but quite hostile.

This case provides a nice example of when we are not able to help. It also points to the need to accept that it is not about our solutions, but rather our being able to ask appropriate and often delving questions. After all, asking the right questions becomes the very means by which the *client* might gain enough insight to be enabled to find the answers s/he has been seeking. At the same time, their answers may clarify for us how we may be able to help.

Ask important questions

Let's begin with a young mother and her four-year-old son, Wing-Li. She was married to a highly motivated professional, and as a family they had moved to this country. Now that they were living in a rural setting, life was so different from their busy city life in Taiwan. Su-Wan admitted she felt ill-equipped to parent her child, having been brought up as an only child largely by an Ama, with little time spent with her own hard-working parents who were highly ambitious for her, their only daughter. But Su-Wan wanted help for her child, believing there was "something wrong with him", believing an early assessment would help her get the best tuition for him before school commenced. She had no friends, so having the active little fellow with her at this first session increased our stress levels, for me and for her.

I was also conscious that my time was costly, so initially I felt constrained by wanting to be most efficient. But the first session basically meant I had to spend most of the time on the floor, playing games with little Wing-Li, while occasionally gaining insights about the family from his mother. This low eye-level focus on the small boy also enabled me to make some general observations of the sharp-eyed little fellow: to observe his capacity to focus, his enjoyment with challenges, and yet his seeming disconnection from his mother. As a mother, she seemed very demanding, even anxiously controlling, never wanting him to make a mistake, nor to do anything that might be deemed (by her) to be unacceptable to me. Gathering information from Su-Wan was also made difficult by some language difficulties, and my own limited experience with her strong Asian accent. Facing my frustrations throughout this session encouraged me to ask her to make a summary in writing before the next session: things that she felt worried about, particularly in terms of her son's behaviours; what things her husband thought to be problems; what she hoped to achieve by seeing me.

Client perception of problem/solution

Having her reflect in writing was a means of helping her clarify to herself what she perceived to be the big issues. Her written report thus provided me with clearer idea of the expectations she held about what might be done for her son, and these helped to expose and then remove any unrealistic presuppositions that I could be held responsible for. In addition, her summary revealed much about her unmet needs, relationally with her husband as well as her son. Her comments exposed the strong resentments she harboured about being taken away from her family of origin. A sense of her isolation clearly demanded real empathy: for her loneliness, her need to be personally affirmed, and also for her perceived significant anxiety about her son. Su-Wan clearly appreciated the expressed concern for her – after all, no one else really knew her needs. But her response, you can imagine, was conflicted: after all, she was not used to expressing her feelings; she was even less likely to have expected personal understanding from a stranger. Eventually her tears brought some relief, but also some embarrassment, with the result that, surprisingly, even her little boy wanted to comfort his mum.

Hidden feelings often shroud hidden needs.

However, my now knowing her real needs did not mean that I personally had to meet them, but rather, my role was to encourage her to find solutions. This included providing some potential contacts within the limited but local centres who were sympathetic to migrant needs, so that some of her needs, like for friendship, could be met. Her summary had also suggested to me that our next discussion could well unleash various hidden emotional needs that she had refused to acknowledge to herself, and certainly had never been expressed to her husband. This meant she needed to come alone, so finding a way for her to have her child minded became important. Gaining her trust was essential to her facing her own needs first, for these had been masked by her focus on her child. Wing-Li had become the reason for her unhappiness, so it was he who had to be fixed! Can you see that some very deep feelings underlay her coming for help? While these remained unacknowledged, the real problems could not be addressed.

It was also interesting to find, over a number of subsequent sessions, that her little boy was really quite bright. In fact, he was not so much in need of an academic assessment, but more in greater need of emotional understanding, evidenced by the reported unacceptable behaviours that suggested being somewhat deprived on that level. Over the following sessions without the child, his mother came to understand that he was reacting massively to his "helicopter" parent, over-restrained, frustrated by his mother's unhealthy demands in her need to control. His normal childish reactions were not understood or accepted, accentuated by her lack of meaningful interactions with other parents, and also by her own feelings of inadequacy as a parent. Even her cultural background became something she needed encouragement to explore. Su-Wan came to a point of realisation that she had little understanding of what she could allow her son to do. For example, she had never taken him to a playpark, believing he might "get germs if he played in the dirt and get sick!".

You may reflect further here on other aspects about her needs that you might find desirable to consider with her.

Unhelpful reactions to strong emotional expressions

At this point, I think it may be helpful to reflect on quite common responses when listening to someone who expresses strong emotions. What do *you* find comes quickly off your tongue when someone shares something that triggers a memory for you? “Oh don’t be upset – you shouldn’t feel like that!” Or alternatively, often we hear responses like: “Oh yes, I know how you feel, ’cos when X happened to me, I felt really Z!” Now, such responses may well be a way of letting the other know you can appreciate their feeling that way. However, too often the focus then shifts to *your* experience, leaving the other feeling deflated by that quick move away from their personal situation. This reduces their opportunity to express their own distressing feelings, while diminishing a belief that the listener really wants to support them. An alternative is needed, one that makes sure you will stay with them while their feelings are explored, to the point where they no longer feel overwhelmed. If your response remains authentic, such as by asking more details of how those feelings are impacting them, this engaging really does wonders for the person.

I remember the many times I experienced feelings of inadequacy after having listened for most of the first session to the pent-up feelings expressed, unsure about where to start with all the issues that had been shared, feeling rather dumped on, and almost emotionally saturated! Then, as the person was leaving, often with an obviously renewed sense of hope that things might get better, he or she (like Su-Wan) would say: “Thank you so much for listening! I feel so much better now”. I had only listened, though was obviously appreciated as one who cares and seems to understand. Variations on this response were often a surprise, particularly when those responses were not made directly to me but to the receptionist while making a further appointment. Don’t be surprised about how often this occurs, when you the listener may be left feeling heavy, with all the implications of the details left with you seeming to impact quite powerfully, *as if* you have been left with having to solve their complex problems!

Our own experiences elicit powerful emotions.

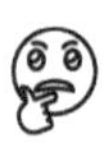 Take some moments now to reflect on other typical responses you may have experienced. How do people generally respond when they have been told about an accident, or a debilitating illness, and may genuinely want to say something to make the other feel better?

Maybe you have heard (or even made) some of these comments: “Oh well, but at least it wasn’t as bad as . . .” Or another: “Yeah awful, but don’t worry, it should improve . . .” Or what about the response: “Yes, I know, but . . . let’s talk about something else, this will help take your mind off . . .!”

Similar typically distractive responses suggest that the listener is self-protecting, to avoid letting the pain of the other become something that impacts personally or too profoundly on the listener. Have you experienced such a fob-off? Or dare I suggest, is it possible that even you may have felt guilty at times about when you used this technique, partly hoping it would help the person move beyond their grief or sadness, without realising it was quite unhelpful?

Catch yourself; honestly reflect on why you would continue to try to minimise the shared feelings of someone who trusts you enough to share their hurts. Whether this sharing occurs between friends or within the context of therapy, appropriate listening will encourage such a level of sharing that brings about potential new light on the grief. But this will never occur if a blind or shutter is pulled down, for such a response in effect only blocks your being recognised as an effective communicator, and your relationship will no longer be valued as trustworthy and caring.

When we listen with integrity, we are clearly saying we *want* to listen. In Chapter 3, however, we will address the very real need to respond when, honestly, we don't want to listen. You may already be thinking about when and where such alternative responses are legitimate, and in fact may be necessary to have in your repertoire of choices. Hang on to these questions until that chapter!

Treating others as we'd like to be treated

How are your reflections going on your own "normal" behaviours? It is much easier to reflect on someone else, isn't it? I have found so often that while questioning others, I too must consider my own behaviours, desiring to be authentic when seeking to support others on the journey. How can I ask others to identify something in themselves that creates a problem, while still masking a similar pattern underlying my own behaviour?

Perhaps we need to ask what makes questioning such a powerful and effective tool. Maybe you think that it is possibly our clever preparations – having a list of good questions that one sticks to like a checklist – that will be important. Is that simply to make sure we now have all the facts?

It was commonly found by students in supervision and in their research involving one-to-one questioning that set questions were deemed to cover all bases. Clearly not, since more information, inevitably, will later be revealed, well after the best series of predetermined questions. We can never anticipate how people will respond; such responses may lead us in unexpected directions, even down serendipitous rabbit holes! But when you reflect on your best interchanges with friends or colleagues, you will recognise that one of you is the good listener! Is that you? You may even find that there are few people who really listen to *you*, and you may wonder why. However, it is a skill that *can* be learned, and will only develop when committed to practice, with an understanding of the related cost involved.

The good listener

Being a good listener is absolutely essential for any engagement that counts between people. This skill demands us to be prepared to put other things aside while we give our absolute attention to what is being communicated. Some of us can do two things at once: ironing while discussing the afternoon's activities is a good example. However, if the one *not* ironing needs to *believe* you are really listening, you may need to down tools!

I am reminded of an only child, Tom (aged eight), given a session with me as a psychologist. He had run away after school, rather than going straight home. Eventually Tom had been found by police some hours later. He seemed unwilling to discuss with anyone why he had run away: with his teachers, the police, or even his Mum, Sharon. Before the session with Tom, Sharon had shared with me how he rarely talked with her, and for some time had seemed to resent any questions about school, about his mates, or what he'd learnt, so she had stopped asking. The school however reported that although he seemed intense in class, Tom always did great work, and was always respectful and cooperative. Do *you* have any hunches about why Tom now failed to explain his running away?

Reflecting on the incident, I recall that it did not take very many minutes alone with Tom to discover his reason. The questions went something like this:

"Tom, you usually go straight home after school, is that right?" He nodded.

I then asked: "And when you get home normally, would you like to tell me what you normally do?" Tom shook his head.

So I continued: "Is that because you wish things were different when you go home?" He nodded again.

"Aha", as I smiled: "I reckon that was because you are always hungry, and your Mum won't give you anything to eat before dinner, am I right?"

"No!" said Tom. "It's because I'm never allowed to go out and play at the dam by myself."

"Oh, that must be very annoying, Tom. You really like playing at the dam, hey?"

"Yes, 'cos I love finding frogs! They are my friends," said Tom.

"Aha . . . and have you always liked frogs, Tom?" He nodded, then said spontaneously: "but Mum said I've got to do my homework first, and then it's always dark, so I can't go outside."

"Oh dear", I said, "that must make you feel really sad, hey Tom?"

"Nah, it just makes me angry. Then Mum bans me for the next week from going to the dam even at the weekend! Then Mum says: 'You're just like your father – he was always angry and look what happened to him!'"

Very quietly I then ask: "Would you like to tell me what happened to him, Tom?"

Tom shook his head. He hung his head and started to cry. We just sat quietly for several minutes, then I asked quietly:

"Did he go away, Tom?" He nodded. "But he used to take you down to the dam, Tom?" Again he nodded.

"So, has Mum ever talked to you about why Dad went away, Tom?" He simply shook his head.

"And you wonder if *you* did something that made him go away, Tom?" Tom nodded again, looking up with a sad face.

"Can you think of anything you did that might have made him go away, Tom?" He shook his head.

"But you really miss him, don't you, Tom?" He quickly nodded, and then said: "He was my best friend – we always talked about a lot of things. Like where frogs come from, and what they eat, and things like that."

Then after some quiet moments, he reflected further on other favourite activities he had enjoyed with his dad. I believed it was time to ask Tom several gently worded questions about how he felt about his mother. Though slow to respond, he finally said he thought she didn't care about him because she never wanted to do things with him.

The discussion went on from there. You may reflect on where it went to next but suffice to say, towards the end of that session, with Tom's approval, I was able to ask his mum to join us. She was then able to hear from Tom what until then he had not been able to clarify to himself, let alone say to his mum, about how badly he was missing his father. Perhaps due to her own grief, and her inability to speak openly to her son about the relationship break-up, her silence had left this introverted but deeply sensitive and thinking small boy sadly creating his own conclusions. These clearly needed to be challenged, but only his mother could do that. She had not been able to share, nor had she even tried to imagine where her child was at. Perhaps you can imagine just why she hadn't – but clearly the child had unwittingly been left alone in his own grief.

Here you will appreciate that *my* natural "parent" feelings needed to be guarded. Yet they also informed me, the psychologist: to listen closely, to really take on board the seriousness of what this child was expressing, indicated further by his withdrawn body language. I needed to stay with where the boy was leading the interchange, treating his comments as his own reality, so that his feelings needed to be explored, regardless of the superficial and apparent facts that may as yet have only partially explained those feelings.

The art of listening – mirroring

> *Are you a good listener? What do you think is the essential element that people respond to the most?*

Surely whether one is a good listener relates to knowing what questions to ask with integrity. But then, crucially, there is the additional demand that the listener really concentrates on understanding the *meaning* behind the answers received. But like with any skill, if we accept the fact that we need to give ourselves time to develop it, we will improve *with practice*, especially if we also give ourselves permission to make mistakes in the learning, which will also bring success!

Reflection implies mirroring: the good listener reflects as closely as possible to what has been heard and understood by the communication, demonstrating thereby a genuine interest. But it is not just the facts that need to be acknowledged, like a parrot; more importantly, it is about the feelings expressed that seem to underlie what was shared. Be prepared to be corrected however, if you get it wrong, just as when I suggested to Tom that he felt sad, but was corrected by his clear "no, I was angry".

The whole nuts and bolts of careful reflection and listening effectively will be discussed in following chapters, as we reflect on other life stories. Such stories will also more fully explore appropriate skills in assertiveness (as compared with aggressive communication), in discovering hidden feelings, and learning to discern the good from the unhelpful questions to ask. But check for yourself now what you have gained from this chapter, then use the following exercises to guide your reflections.

REVISION EXERCISES

- The question of motivation was a necessary consideration in the decision to write this book. As referred to in the foreword, desiring to pass on to others what has been learned over many years of practice is the main motivator here. What is *your* motivation, even for why you are reading this book? Do you simply want someone to answer your questions, so you will have answers to give away?
- Are you seriously hoping you'll learn more about yourself? Perhaps you want to learn how others think, hear what others have experienced, and so grow in self-understanding that you may improve your interactions with others.

Remain conscious of the motivation that drives you: challenge the need to be successful, or to never let someone go without fixing their problem. If your motivation is really wanting to know how to better help people – a worthy motivator held by many interested in psychology – then briefly summarise the questions or statements you may now want to practise, even as you reflect on yourself and how you would answer in response to someone genuinely needing to hear your answers. You may also find it useful to create a long list of potential conversation starters that enable others to open up about themselves.

> *"Why" is often not a good question to ask!*

It is important to realise that in asking Why, you should *expect* a rational, reasonable response. But if there are strong emotions still brewing, perhaps even not yet recognised or acknowledged, rational understandings are not going to be readily available or forthcoming. You will be given *some* explanations because you've asked for them, but rarely will these provide the real reason for the action, belief or attitude.

Asking the right questions is so important, to encourage people to consider what the potential answers reveal about *themselves*: Tell me something about yourself . . . or, what do you think might be . . . or, *how* does it make you feel about . . . *when* do find yourself doing . . . or, can you share with me times when the people in your life did . . . and *what* made you feel . . . Questions of What, How, and When are much more likely to reveal the truth about what was experienced by the client, particularly until the powerful emotional elements are confronted and explored, with genuine warmth, understanding, and acceptance.

When people open up to exploring answers to these questions, you will inevitably experience the satisfaction of many clients – like Su-Wan mentioned earlier – saying: "Thank you so much for helping me. I'm now feeling up to facing some things I couldn't face before coming here." You know you have simply asked lots of genuine, concerned, and caring questions, and then affirmed your client's personal but thoughtful reflections! Their various answers may then be questioned further, with the client often reflecting with "I'd never thought to ask myself that." Such teasing out of the answers given often enables clients to find possible solutions for themselves.

> *Be honest: how well do you really listen?*
> *Check out what your best friend thinks about you as a listener.*

Chapter 2

Reflections that highlight the real issue

This chapter seeks to identify specific problems that may create blockages to effective communications between the helper and the helped. These include clearly identifying the focus of the problem brought for attention, and how the purposeful use of reflection during relaxation may minimise unnecessary or awkward reactions. Examples include emotions that call for empathy, yet when clarified may require different responses than those you would normally express. Other issues are identified that may create a lack of trust, suggested by a limited insight into others' perceived depth of feelings, often due to but not limited by cultural or familial differences. Personal growth is encouraged, with reflective listening highlighted as an essential.

As we begin this journey, I'd like you to stop and imagine a favourite picture: one in which reflection is beautifully obvious. Is your picture at the beach, over a lake, perhaps, with silhouettes of a boat or trees, or with a magnificent sunrise or sunset? The clearer the elements of reflection are, the same beautiful picture will be seen even if turned upside down! Sit now with your imagined picture: enjoy the associated feelings.

Reflection itself is fundamental in just about everything we do. Apart from the value of putting that experience or new understanding into longer-term memory, good reflection is essential – not just for the enjoyment received from the visuals, but also for ensuring accurate perception of the message received. Sometimes we are guilty of giving very unclear messages, and these remain so unless someone dares to ask: "What did you mean?" Without honest self-reflection, before, during, and after completion of a task or a message we want to send or have received, we risk missing the crucial components of its meaning or worthwhileness. Our common quick potential miscommunications of SMS messages provide good examples of what can happen if we don't check and reflect, before sending!

Reflection

Without reflection, we may risk an unwitting repetition of unwise or even inappropriate actions. We may also fail to effectively confront the very

DOI: 10.4324/9781003474746-2

expectations we want to achieve over those things which continue to disappoint us. How often do you normally take time out to engage in reflecting on your life? Do you ever challenge yourself to be more alert to any patterns of behaviour in yourself that may be less than helpful?

It may help to recall how reflections are also appropriate for effectively working with others, assisting us in knowing what the real issues are. In the case of Su-Wan mentioned in our first chapter, you will remember that while she perceived her son Wing-Li had a problem, close examination of the issues meant that the real problems lay more at *her* feet than at her child's. Identification of these altered the direction of possible future solutions.

But let's return to another case which demonstrates that, so often, the perceived problem that a person presents with can be very different from the one finally understood as the main issue. Such awareness requires wise reflective questioning around the mixture of feelings and facts, along with their responses.

Identification of real issues versus presenting problems

Sam, a serious man in his early forties, claimed that he wanted help to know how to resolve his guilt over planning to leave his wife. He said he was really depressed, and this he acknowledged made all the family unhappy. So, being no longer in love with his wife, he felt he should leave her and his children – but, he sadly admitted, he felt terribly guilty about this option. Sam considered himself to be usually conscientious, about everything, and was clearly not comfortable with his present reaction. There was no one else in the picture, and yet getting away seemed so desirable, so impelling, even to be inevitable.

Through my persistent and quiet questioning, he gradually came to realise that he had always ignored his feelings, now clearly identified, as he recalled repressing all feelings throughout his unhappy childhood. This realisation enabled him to reflect on his childhood reaction to the frequent anger expressed violently between parents, their frightening discord which had eventually caused them to separate. He had early formed a strong belief: emotions were best bottled, so that he had become completely committed to the belief that *all* confrontations needed to be avoided.

Perhaps here you can reflect on what impact this may have had on his current relationships, particularly with his wife, but also towards their growing children. Further questions brought him to a surprising revelation: his commitment to non-confrontation had also had dire implications for how he functioned at work. Sam finally admitted that, for him, work was awful: there were so many issues he could not deal with because he feared that with confronting them came the potential for anger.

Questions that reflect on benefits of maintaining personal beliefs

Here you may imagine how questioning the benefits of holding such definite views needed careful understanding. The process of guided reflections allowed Sam to get to a point where he could discuss with me how some people he knew and respected had happily maintained good relationships, even when daring to frequently argue. Arguments, putting one's views even quite strongly, started to look like being potentially a healthy part of daily life. New potentials then became possibilities to be considered.

He was also encouraged to wonder how he might feel should he simply write down the problems seen at work. He agreed to try this, and carefully produced a great page at his next session! Within the ensuing discussions he began to grasp the enormity of workplace problems. He reported being bullied, used, and often scapegoated, since he was well known to never fire up in self-defence.

But he also mentioned inner turmoil, often feeling conflicted about several moral issues around tasks he was responsible for, but which he couldn't dare confront. He visibly gained some relief just having shared these. He was, understandably, quite surprised by his very mixed feelings when his own perceptions were clarified and validated.

It was then my privilege to affirm such conflicting feelings, with my understanding of why these might be so disturbing for him. This meant I could safely posit the possibility that such work issues might potentially be the greater source of his unhappiness, rather than his marriage. He then became open to the process of questioning not only his long-held belief that "silence is golden", but also, by maintaining this attitude, the unhappy implications on the very people who really mattered. It had become evident to him, at home and even more so at work, that silence was an ineffective and problematic way to keep the peace.

> *Correct focus enables clarity about possible solutions.*

Challenges for Sam thus were on several fronts: from his firmly held beliefs about disagreements, established as a child, his learning to confront matters in a respectful way inevitably revealed issues both at the personal level as well as at work. This process involved teaching and demonstration concerning the differences between being passive or non-assertive and being aggressive, and a constructive alternative to both of these: the rich, newly empowering concept of being assertive. More on these styles of communication a little later.

Modelling and teaching these skills needed to be handled with care, so that educating him did not create resentment towards his ill-equipped parents; rather, it aimed to provide him with a greater and empowering understanding, which he acknowledged had not been available to his parents. Understanding is one thing, but changing behaviour requires *experiencing* real alternatives.

Role-playing enables new behaviours

This new way of thinking thus involved engaging Sam in a number of role-plays with me, to practise and experience how best to confront various situations, with real-life examples. Confronting bothersome issues involved my role-playing various relationships, such as his wife, boss or other work colleague. Role-playing provides a context for the practice needed to enable newly informed intentions to become part of anyone's behavioural repertoire. With this came greater confidence for Sam to believe in his capability to overcome his old reluctance to address conflicts.

Even after making some good relational changes, Sam then faced some bigger issues that eventually he needed to share with his wife. In his workplace he found bosses to be set against trying to find solutions that might cost them financially – for example, accepting the need to hire extra employees, or making time for discussions that were not high on the employers' priorities. In the end, the options for many facing such dilemmas involve rethinking whether or not to stay in such employment, or to seek support from legal entities concerning one's rights.

In this case study alone, our attention is brought to necessary communications that are frequently delivered with considerable emotions. When this occurs, we need ways of handling these with a sensitivity that does not cause the other either to be embarrassed about what the open communications have revealed, or to become very angry because of it. On the other hand, if *we* personally feel awkward about handling another's strong reactions that are seemingly over the top, imagine what stress that can put the *client* under, resulting perhaps in the client wishing to leave the uncomfortable situation. Should that person quit such an interchange, however, do not beat yourself up. You will have become more aware, and your sincere and honest self-reflection afterwards will enable you to learn another good lesson!

> *Expressed emotions can create awkward situations.*

So, how do we react to the client who shares some disturbing feelings about an event in their life and in so doing becomes visibly upset and seemingly embarrassed? You may quite naturally wish to comfort, give a hug, rush in with tissues, or even become upset yourself. Between friends, such reactions are considered normal, but in a more clinical setting, any of these responses can be inappropriate, making it difficult for you to think what to say or do next to cover embarrassment all round. Even saying 'I know how you feel' is also so often inappropriate and unhelpful – clients may rightly believe you really *can't* know what they are feeling!

Can you suggest what else may be an effective response, one that allows you to demonstrate care without becoming overwhelmed? What would you do when a client, like little Tom for example, finally admits with tears that he really misses his dad? Likewise, what would you do with Su-Wan, when she finally admits with tears how inadequate she feels as a migrant parent?

Alternatives may readily come to mind. While sensitively and quietly you would offer the tissue box, hopefully you would consider it appropriate to just sit quietly, while the person's tears flow, before reassuring him or her with some comment like "it is so good to be able to let feelings out, isn't it", or "you know, there is no reason to feel in any way embarrassed about your feelings; I am honoured that you trust me in sharing these important reactions with me." And eventually, you may find it appropriate to remark: "I hope you understand how important it is to let our feelings out. This means we can move on from them, when we are not trapped by those feelings."

It is also valuable for a client or hurting person to know how important it is to share feelings, both in a safe place and with someone they know who cares. The person may still find their emotional outburst difficult to deal with; you will have seen some who apologise for letting you see their distress. So, some analogies may be important to share, supported by the more physiological understanding they already know, like how wonderful pain relief is after medication, or when a painful abscess finally bursts. Another analogy may also provide reassurance, when reference is made to how crippling fear can be until that fear is appropriately dismissed, and replaced with a far healthier understanding that in itself brings relief.

This briefly brings us to another important consideration: Empathy. How important is this in your own relationships?

Appropriate empathy – but understand transference

Empathy is often considered an essential if we are to help people in need. However, it can also be an Achilles' heel, particularly for the person who too quickly is driven by feelings. Are you perhaps that someone? Just like the discomfort of trying to wear someone else's shoes, too much entering into another's pain can become the very thing that prevents you from seeing the real issues, and therefore inhibits your capacity to do what you set out to do – to clarify the problem while supporting the sufferer.

For example: imagine a person shares a disturbing dilemma with you. That person has fallen in love with another person while already in a seemingly good and healthy marriage or relationship. If *you* are personally experiencing similar conflicting feelings, or have been hurt by another in the past, unless you can disassociate from those feelings (and have formed a healthy personal conclusion to your own story), you may lead the other into wrong decisions about their own potential future actions. You may also know stories of some who have lapsed in their commitment to maintaining objective relations in counselling. Having become too emotionally involved with their client, some have taken inappropriate actions that in the end become damaging for both carer and client, though with the best of intentions.

Are your *own* feelings likely to get in the way? Check out your understanding of transference and countertransference. Don't become caught out by ignorance about how powerfully these both can influence the outcomes. Confront where your own feelings originate from. Learn to share these with another understanding trusted person, so that your experience and its associated feelings need no longer dominate your own perceptions. Feelings are powerful and when positive can be wonderful. But they can considerably distort the facts – like when we experience not being able to see the wood for the trees – and can become detrimental of a positive way forward.

Feelings can get in the way.

Feelings are naturally occurring reactions to events or circumstances, which erupt as human emotions. Quite often, these are simply visceral or body responses that we can't control. For example, the visceral responses in those of us who admit to hating heights can be so enormously powerful that we perspire profusely, heartbeats go crazy, and we find it impossible to finish or even to attempt the climb ahead. Many feelings seem equally uncontrollable – like being annoyed by a neighbour's persistent barking dog or angry at a person who steals your parking spot. More seriously, feelings of despair when nothing seems to go right can be so crushing, so debilitating. However, what we do with those feelings becomes the critical part: first step, are *you* able to acknowledge these to yourself? And, when appropriate, do you share these with another who cares about how you feel? Do you understand how this sharing goes a long way to resolving the issue, especially when freed from the pressing power of the underlying masked feelings that had so debilitated you?

How well do you appropriately explore hidden feelings?

Remember the first client mentioned, Su-Wan (Chapter 1), and how her own unmet needs were ignored, creating a perceived problem with her child.

Now reflect on what happens to you when you have not eaten breakfast, and the workplace expects you to forgo an early lunch to attend a compulsory staff meeting – your need for energising food unwittingly escalates into anger at the boss. Or think of how your own feelings towards a friend may change dramatically when you hear a bit of gossip supposedly shared by that same friend about you that was not true. In this case, acknowledging your emotions can be so important. Doing so is not just about confronting the truth, but also creating the potential to learn more about the basis of your friendship. It can prevent you from wrongly concluding that no one is to be trusted.

Submissive, aggressive versus assertive communications

There are important distinctions that need to be made about how people express feelings, and this appropriately involves understanding the important difference between offering submissive, aggressive, or assertive communications. Often being a submissive "yes person" is simply born out of a drive to keep the peace, while an aggressive person simply shares strong feelings without any concern for who or what is affected, thus destroying good relations. Interestingly, in the long run, submissiveness doesn't make for good relationships either as it eventually creates resentment, and often is finally demonstrated by being passively aggressive.

Rather than resorting to the first two options, we find that learning to be more assertive brings about a healthy style of honest communications, enabling you to be more appropriately able to say how you feel, while being respectful of others. Any of these three patterns may have been adopted because of family or cultural expectations, however, and we will review these more fully with other client cases in later chapters.

For the moment, however, even in relation to Su-Wan, you may reflect on cultural differences that would naturally have affected her understanding of her difficulties. But remember that these are not only observed between different ethnic groups of people, but also between families, where certain historical patterns of behaviour are modelled and thought to either be acceptable or as "can't be helped"!

Be aware of cultural differences

For some people, as initially observed with Sam in relation to beliefs about people in his family, such differences may be held to be non-negotiable. We do know that even within families, there can be a particular "culture" that is not appreciated by others from a very different background. Family cultures can be covertly dominated by economic, social, or even religious attitudes and beliefs.

However, gentle questioning can lead a person to reflect, even to challenge their underlying beliefs, to discern the impact of maintaining such when trying to relate to others from a different "culture". This may be also experienced at a sub-cultural level, like intra-family confrontations. Even an individual's beliefs unless modified can form the basis of that person's inability to deal with the presenting problem.

At times being unable to resolve an issue may involve another person, like the partner. A joint consideration of the issue expressed may enable each person to reconsider the benefits of change, as opposed to remaining obdurate. Unless both are involved in this process, the lasting effects of strongly held beliefs and negatively associated feelings will remain problematic in the relationship.

Do you hold any views that are intractable? Be clear about why these may or may not be sacrosanct or non-negotiable.

Feelings that control our cognitions

In Sam's case, after he had acknowledged past hurts and ill-formed beliefs, the learning of how to express ideas and feelings more appropriately allowed him to learn to be more assertive at work about his unmet needs. This did not mean, however, that he was able to change the workplace ideology. A realistic assessment eventually necessitated his finding new employment, and this provided a positive way forward, for him as an individual, and also relationally within his marriage and family. This skill can be seen played out in more detail in the chapter which looks at problem solving.

Grow your understanding

How keenly have you become aware of what good listening is really about? Reflect now on your own ability to sit with another's discussion: do you find yourself mirroring back facts only, without the associated feelings? Are you prepared to risk getting these wrong, so the other can correct you, 'see' what the other is sharing with you? It will mean you need to polish your mirroring back of what you think you have heard. Getting a clear image involves the time to understand, explore, and appreciate the emotions that being a good mirror can reveal. Don't ever think the precious time spent here is ever wasted.

We know what cloudy mirrors are like, but how good it is when they are really clean, especially when we *want* to see what is really there! Reflect again about young Tom: no one had spent enough quality time with him to try to understand what he might be feeling. Or do you, perhaps like Sam, try to ignore feelings, decide you are not going to focus on them, in case doing so will simply amplify the problem? If so, you are not alone in believing feelings should be kept under wraps. But can you see what happened when Tom's feelings were finally drawn out? His knowing that someone seemed to understand him – simply by affirming his emotional needs – was sufficient to engage him in the process of sharing his inner conflicts, which had earlier resulted in his running away.

REVISION EXERCISES

- In each of the cases we've looked at here, I wonder if you recognise any aspect that you personally feel may need to be strengthened.
- Check it with your best friend, or someone you confide in. Facing potential *weaknesses* in yourself is a great first step in reflective practice – and it needs to continue!

In the following chapters, I will be sharing with you more examples of the different issues that people need encouragement to confront. But *you* need to consider how you might use these personal insights, particularly as you continue to learn how to sharpen your intention to be a more astute and effective listener. You will also be asked to honestly reflect on your own *strengths*, as you consider what you might have done differently in the cases referred to.

Chapter 3

How well do we listen?

While we may agree with the importance of listening, sometimes we are not always clear about how best to respond. Self-reflection enables a better understanding that extends to our reading of body language: a different story that can amplify or contradict the words we hear. Good listening invokes supportive language, but at times may also demand action. However, there are times when listening needs to be taught as a skill that is optional, even identified as appropriate or not, depending on interest and availability of time. Keeping good reflective records, supported by good supervision or trustworthy accountability, is considered essential, with practice exercises encouraged that are based on presented client stories.

Can you remember asking or hearing the angry question, "Did you hear me?" What was the reply? Nothing? Or was it simply: "Yes, I heard you!"? Was that the end of the story? It rarely is!

I remember listening to a lady who poured out the sad story of her life, leading me to wonder with some confusion: 'where do I begin to focus my attention?' Her tale was complex and disturbing. It had occupied all of my first hour as I basically listened to her, with little need to ask any questions. I remember thinking that this was not going to be an easy journey. Karena's initial outpouring of grief surrounded her anger at her ex-husband, experienced more particularly after her telling him she could not cope with his lies any longer. When his extra-marital affairs were finally admitted to, he had moved out, rather unwillingly, but after leaving he made clear his intention to make life difficult for her.

The whole story can be quite disturbing, so I will only give details sufficient to explain what tools were needed. It is noteworthy to remember that any information received may not be the whole story.

Karena seemed so deeply disillusioned by her broken marriage to Brett that I just listened, giving minimal comments to indicate I really felt for her. But then I learned she had already been married before, a somewhat abusive relationship. From this, she had a teenage son with whom she reported having a good relationship.

DOI: 10.4324/9781003474746-3

She had expected that this second marriage would simply be better. Initially Brett had provided more than adequately for their finances, with a good house; this quelled her fear of becoming homeless again, as had happened after the first break-up.

However, after learning she was pregnant with their child Delia, Brett had become totally disinterested in her, physically and emotionally. During the pregnancy, she had tried to make new friends, but Brett increasingly became paranoid, accusing her of being unfaithful. He had insisted on her always staying at home, on-call at any time.

Finally Karena found out from some of her friends that Brett had a reputation in the district for being "good with the ladies" – that *he* had left behind a number of shattered relationships, and was locally known as having a history of simply moving on, from one to the next! Now he had indeed moved on from her, leaving her to raise their child not only unsupported, but he also continued to threaten their future well-being. He refused any financial support, either for their child or for such things as payment for car repairs. In any contact he was inevitably aggressive, and in various indirect ways he continued to frustrate her ability to leave her home. Ever conscious of his previous violent and controlling temper, she was fearful of asking for any help, even simply to support their daughter.

Listening to stories of abuse

Naturally, Karena's emotional state at the first interview was such that she needed many pauses to allow her to cry, before she launched into another and often more disturbing aspect of her situation. My listening involved many quiet "oh dears" and "that must have been terrible", but Karena needed little encouragement to keep her story alive. The box of tissues quietly placed next to her gave her permission to be as upset as she needed to be. It is important to note here that listening intently, both to the facts and the emotional import attached to these, can be personally quite draining for the listener too. But I knew that until she had vented the complete story, there was no way that I could discern what her actual needs were. I simply needed to be patient, without judgement or leaping to conclusions. This was not a time to ask her directly as to why she had come.

Effective listening requires reflecting feelings first.

It seemed to take almost the entire session before I was able to hear what I believed to be the crux of her story. This concerned what she should do to stop her three-year-old daughter having to go to her father for the compulsory access visits each month. These she reported had begun only recently, following a court ruling that had insisted the father should regularly see his daughter.

Before leaving Karena, Brett had shown no interest in little Delia. In fact, Karena had thought the separation would be reasonably stress-free, and indeed had been for many months. She then learned that Brett had a new girlfriend who had apparently been surprised that he did not see his daughter. The story the girlfriend had been told was that access had been denied – reportedly Brett excelled at making himself look good socially. Legal demands were then made with which Karena had initially just complied, hoping Brett was now in a better place to be a good father.

However, only after two visits, Delia's behaviour had suddenly changed. She had been completely toilet-trained prior to access, but a year on, at three years old, Delia had suddenly reverted to serious bedwetting. This was also accompanied by disturbing dribbling when she tried to speak. This once happy little girl now reportedly was easily upset, and each time an access visit was mentioned, she withdrew, stubbornly resisting any move towards going.

Initially Karena had simply insisted, delivering a crying, screaming child to her father. This was understandably terribly upsetting for Karena too, but she believed she had no choice. Karena had finally decided to get help when further symptoms of age regression appeared: Delia suddenly would no longer talk, not even with her mother, and eye contact had also become almost non-existent.

Personal reflections that demonstrate understanding

At this point, my role changed: it was not merely to affirm how awful life must be for her. Nor was it adequate to simply ask questions that might stimulate her into finding alternative solutions for herself. It was apparent that a vulnerable child's life was potentially being affected in a way that suggested the possibility of abuse of one kind or other.

An alternative perspective was necessary to assess the truth of her story. It was clear that she loved her daughter and was prepared to do anything that might help. She willingly provided the opportunity for me to speak with Delia, knowing this would not be a one-off occasion. I encouraged her to find financial support for this through a care plan, available at that time through her GP. This made it possible for me to spend a number of short sessions with Delia alone, followed by regular interviews with Karena while Delia played in the waiting room.

Reflection that incites necessary action

To cut a very long story short, I mention here only some of the tools needed over a period of some months. Karena was encouraged to accurately keep a diary of

Delia's various observable behaviours. Gradually Delia became less anxious in sessions with me, as we initially played games with animals, with tiny characters she could action for any imaginary story. I then encouraged her to draw, firstly fun pictures, then later include figurines to help act out her drawings. You will understand that eventually she was asked to draw other things: home, people she loved, then any animals or characters she feared.

Care had to be made not to suggest any ideas that she would just go along with. But her drawings were clear enough, as in session she became more able to express herself, clearly describing what her pictures were about. Disturbingly, her father was never in the picture of the family – until towards the end of four months, when he was angrily drawn in: as a monster.

Observe and record body language

Note must be made here that listening is always interwoven with observing the one speaking: being able to identify body language that changes when describing events or people; legs crossing, arms folding, and the body turned away; watching how the person's eyes become distant or detached, sad, angry, or even excited. These last indicators of underlying feelings about what has been shared will mean we need to check any interpretations with the person concerned. Specific questions would be asked like "I see that excites you – does it make you happy when you think about . . .?". Watch for the head shakes or nods, before offering any alternative understanding. Such questions are kept simple with a small child, but of course with more articulate people, we will more likely include statements like "tell me how that makes you feel . . ." or "can you describe more about that, so I know what you mean".

So, I hear you wondering: what was the end of their story? What was achieved, both for the distressed mother, and for the little girl?

There is not always a good ending, but in this case, I can say that Karena started to feel some relief, knowing that at least her perceptions about things being really bad for her little daughter were being taken seriously. This also gave her more confidence to seek company with other friends. They encouraged her to believe in herself as a parent, and more confidently question and to assert her right to stop Delia's enforced access visits with her father. Initially these were simply curtailed for health reasons, by regularly maintaining Delia was unwell.

Over those several months of non-access, with Karena fearful of being taken to court for refusing to hand over Delia for access visits, the evidence became more compelling: Delia's speech returned and with reduced dribbling; her bedwetting stopped, and finally she clearly was able to say that she never wanted to see her father again. Using her play characters, she was even able to demonstrate some of the sexually revolting things her father expected her to do – impossible for a child so young to create such a heinous picture. Clearly, such ideas were not gained from her mother either.

Be prepared to take supportive action

My understanding of the issues was personally quite disturbing. My discernment of physical and sexual abuse explained the apparent reason why this small vulnerable child had so regressed into being a baby again, with a likely long-term hideous impact on her unless further action was taken.

In all of this I had ascertained that Karena's sense of being disempowered and hopeless had been linked with the ex-husband being part of a wealthy, well-known, and influential local family. With Karena's permission, I wrote a report of my findings to a solicitor well known for defending cases involving sexual assault. His practice was in a large city some considerable distance away. This was done because Karena held little trust in the local rural community, given the small-town issues of everyone knowing who the important people are and who should not be upset. Thankfully for this vulnerable mum and her daughter, the solicitor took the case seriously, and pro bono. Access by the father was finally and decidedly denied by the court. Great relief was apparent for both Karena and her family, and this was certainly my experience, after months of concern for their future!

At my last interview with Karena many months later, Delia had mostly returned to her happy self, now chatting more freely with her mum and happily attending kindergarten. In addition, her teenage brother came in to report, thankfully, on how well his little sister was now doing.

Are you up for another story about listening? Take a break if you need to. Hearing such stories can be quite disturbing, even overwhelming.

This next story is quite different, however, as it involved voluntary adults: a mother and her three adult daughters. The mother, Martha, initially came saying that she was feeling incredibly sad and lonely, because her adult daughters never came to see her. She could not work out what to do.

Her late husband Geoff (the daughters' father) had died after a prolonged illness. Then, soon after his death, she had reconnected with a man she had previously known, and he had moved in with her. Barry had also been recently widowed.

In listening to her story, it was clear that communication within the family had never been their strength. Rather, they reported always being busy, active women, with little time given to sitting and talking. But during Geoff's lengthy illness, Martha had become more reflective, so much so that since his death she had spent much time alone, trying to work out why "her girls" now never visited.

After I listened to her grief – the loss of her husband and more particularly the loss of her girls – my questions flowed into reflecting with her about her new relationship, and what it meant to her. The positive elements expressed about her friend Barry were always interspersed with stronger negative feelings of regret about her girls. This naturally posed questions about what her daughters might be feeling about the loss of their father, and what they might have been thinking about his replacement.

It was surprising to me that someone of her age (early 60s) had never thought about matters from any other point of view but her own. But it was also a significant move for her now to have sought help, and I wondered why. That question brought fresh insights, for it was the new man in her life who had insisted she get help. Barry had suggested to her that it was unlikely their relationship would last unless things were sorted, saying he couldn't abide her negative moods.

Of course, when such feelings are raised, most people need permission to vent them, and this is never easy for someone whose normal manner is to repress such feelings, keeping them concealed, both from oneself and from others. It is always tricky to move such a discussion into the more emotional zone, and some people need to go away to think about and explore such feelings on their own before another help session. This proved to be the case with Martha, so she was warned that she might feel quite down, facing many things in that week. However, I encouraged her to understand that even writing such feelings down would bring some relief to her pent-up, unexpressed feelings. I also suggested that she try to share some of her insights with Barry, asking for his patience.

Encourage reflections with others in relationships

In the following meeting with Martha, it was reassuring to hear that she was already feeling a little less despondent. Barry had been more understanding than she had expected. So now she was eager to consider ways that might bring about some connection with her daughters. She had reflected on their lack of communication with her, on many levels, and was inclined to blame herself. This provided a good opening, asking about family patterns over the years, and naturally encouraged her to consider differences she had observed about her girls when they were growing up – using such questions like "did any of the girls seem more like their Dad?" and "describe how they each were at home, with each other" and "How were they different at school?".

When you encourage such reflections from people of any age, you will often hear their surprise expressed at remembered circumstances, as they are provided with a new and surprising understanding of earlier events that had been completely forgotten. Sometimes such understanding is not easily assimilated into a later context, which often prevents a greater appreciation of why others behave as they do. Listening in this context involves affirming the previous knowledge, and helping people see the current connections lost with time. Some of this understanding is assisted by talking about individual differences and personality – but more of this later in Chapters 12 and 13.

Expect to hear raw emotions – not always rational

I'd like to conclude briefly here on how this case was resolved. At my instigation, each of the adult (30-plus) daughters was invited to attend with their mother, having simply been told that she was needing their help. She half-expected they would decline, but they all did arrive, obviously concerned. My listening skills were second only to the importance of asking some caring but important *questions* of where each was at, while at the same time, I knew they were all obviously curious, eager to understand why they were there. Of these quiet but confident women, it only took the one more emotionally in tune with her mother to start their discussion. Clearly, they were not used to sharing feelings, but there was no doubt about the fact that they cared for her. Hearing such positive statements was quite important and brought ready tears from Martha. It was also necessary that questions of how they felt about losing their father were differently explored with each, so that Martha more clearly came to understand how each was indeed grieving. This helped to somewhat explain their infrequent visits, each of them not wanting to add further to their mother's distress.

However, I remember one of the daughters openly expressed some anger at how quickly Barry had been allowed to move in. This was a complete surprise to Martha, and potentially looked like it would undo some of the positive interchanges just begun together. But it is important to note here that appropriate listening needs to include mirroring reflections, to clarify what is being expressed. Some of these for you to think about include: "So am I right in hearing you really felt angry towards . . . because of . . .?" Or "Did the decision made by your Mum mean you felt . . .?", "and did this mean you decided not to visit often, in case . . .?" Or maybe, "What would you like to say to your Mum about how you felt? Do you still feel angry . . . or perhaps after hearing more from Mum today about her feelings, is there another feeling you may want her to know about now?" It naturally flowed on into the *four* women each feeling free to engage in a crossflow of thoughts and feelings, as I remained aware of the need to safely diffuse potential misunderstandings.

Questions to clarify feelings

Teasing out the meanings of expressed feelings is so incredibly helpful. After all, you will appreciate that so often feelings can distort, exaggerate, or even confuse the real issues that are causing us to behave in certain ways. For instance, if we are feeling sad and can't express that publicly for fear of breaking down emotionally, then defensively we seek to find other reasons for why we behave the way we do, thereby excusing or justifying our actions. This is what we mean when we say someone has resorted to *rationalising* their responsive behaviour. It may also be helpful to think about feelings as being like the tip of an iceberg – the real power and the depth of the feelings "under the water" are far more important for understanding what is going on.

Strong feelings are analogous to an iceberg.

Perhaps you can now see how Barry, the man who unwittingly was seen to have taken their father's place, became the unexpressed but considered *real* reasoning for why the grieving daughters had neglected their mother. Such conclusions, however, always need to be checked – and in this case, that reasoning had been true for two of the women, and an open discussion ensued between Martha and two of her caring but hurting daughters.

The third daughter expressed genuine sorrow at having neglected her Mum. Finally, each daughter openly admitted to her own personal needs that had taken up most of their time and energy. Again, this explanation brought more tears, tears of relief as well as sadness, while creating a very real opportunity for developing greater closeness.

To summarise this chapter on listening, particularly if the things to be shared are likely to have deep or serious repercussions, I'd like to make three cautionary points:

1. Listening needs to indicate a *genuine* interest in what is to be shared.
2. Unless one has the time and emotional energy to give *at that moment*, it is far better to arrange the earliest but agreed *future* time, rather than risk a rushed interchange that becomes incomplete/unsatisfying for either party.
3. Listening will often mean your own feelings may be aroused, and unless you know what to do with *these* feelings, any attempt to resolve an issue with someone else may become convoluted, and potentially quite destructive.

So the next chapter will focus on what we need to understand about our own vulnerabilities, our own inclination to be reactive, as well as how we need to be thoughtfully prepared. This knowledge should enable us to strengthen our desire to improve relationships, rather than retreat from them. Such personal honesty helps prevent the war of words that can inevitably mean we wished the issues were treated as sleeping dogs – best left alone.

REVISION EXERCISES

1. Seriously reflect now on each of the cases mentioned in this chapter: reread them, and even write a summary of what you now understand about listening.
2. Consider what you might have done in each example if you had been involved with a similar person and their needs.
3. Now reflect on your own listening skills: how did you go this week? Were there occasions when you did well, or wished you'd done better? Perhaps you found listening with genuine concern really difficult, especially when you were asked to listen to something in which you have little interest.
4. What were you meant to say or do differently in such instances? Write down some options, so that you can be prepared next time.

Read on! You may gain some helpful insights in the next chapter. And remember the old adage: s/he who makes no mistakes makes nothing!

Chapter 4

What to do when listening is tough?

Further reflections on how tough listening can be warrants being more aware of the implications of emotions that can distort future outcomes. Be this from the power of self-talk, or the power of disturbing experiences that leave heavy marks, associated feelings can frequently be lost, covered over with irrational beliefs that need to be unearthed. Specific problems, often reported as blame of others, will be demonstrably manageable when identified by "who owns the problem". These problems can then best be resolved when understanding the valuable differences possible when using "I-messages or statements" as a means of sending an acceptable message as opposed to "You-messages/ statements". Problem ownership also teaches how effective listening becomes an essential component in problem solving. Such knowledge is effective only with much practice, which the Reflective Exercises encourage.

We really like to think of ourselves as approachable, caring people, don't we? We like to believe we always make the time to listen whenever there is a genuine need. But really, if we are honest, this is a big ask for anyone, isn't it? After all, we are human, we are not God, and our personal needs surely mean some boundaries are necessary – essential if we are to protect ourselves from burnout! We simply cannot risk finishing up crashing in a burnt-out heap of resentment, feeling used, and taken for granted. How do we rightly manage this, so that we are not seen to be selfish, uncaring people?

This frequently experienced dilemma about how we care for ourselves while caring too greatly about others will also be looked at in Chapter 18, Caring for the Carer. But let's briefly reflect here on the places where you would anticipate such an issue to be experienced.

You will recognise that workplaces, especially those providing human support services, present the most common situations in which people *feel* they should act unselfishly, and too often with little gratitude ever expressed in return. Think of schools, hospitals – nurses, doctors, cleaners, counsellors, social workers, clergy, lawyers, shops, the building industry, or even those administratively working for a company. Indeed, are there *any* occupations where conscientious individuals are

DOI: 10.4324/9781003474746-4

not likely to suffer from this problem? Yes, you may say, the people who work for themselves. Really? What about parents – and, sometimes, the grandparents of today's busy world? Maybe this issue is rife, even if they have no other relationships which demand their attention. These examples alone may help us see why we often find ourselves listening to people who have periodically if not permanently withdrawn from close relationships, in order to protect themselves. But at some point, most of us face the need to find ways of deciding where our personal priority lies – where giving becomes muddied with the need to look after oneself.

How to care for myself while caring for others?

Ok, let's think about what you might typically do when you are racing off to work, and someone calls you up, clearly expressing strong feelings about an issue that you might also care about. What do you normally do? Choose to be late, and risk being reprimanded, yet again? Or do you get so anxious that your own feelings become confused, and you say some things you later wished you'd not said? Or perhaps you tell the caller you haven't time just now – maybe you'll contact them later, when you've time, but you never do. And what about that email: one that contains something you know is important to the writer, and although you care about them, right now you really don't give a . . . about this current issue. Do you think about what to say, but don't even bother to reply? Or choose to just forget it, as too hard to deal with?

Feeling guilty? Or just uncomfortable?

Take a few minutes here to consider honestly what your typical personal response is to the frequent demands on your time and interest. You may sometimes regret how you acted, how you gave in and, yet again, simply said Yes. You may be surprised to realise you *did* have choices. However, it is always much easier to say Yes to someone, rather than No, especially when that would mean feeling terrible about letting someone down.

Should I always be available?

In my personal need to reflect on this question, someone else immediately comes to mind: James, who was the pastor of a growing church, in a somewhat challenged community. There were so many needs, and he believed he should conscientiously try to meet as many as possible. After all, James enthusiastically went into this job with a clear call to service. He sought to sincerely reflect his great spiritual Master whom history has recognised as having given his all. In his first session, while pouring out where he was at, however, James expressed the wish to right now be working someplace else: a place where he imagined he could regain a once-experienced sense of joy and peace.

He also admitted he felt very guilty because others who had been joining him for some time had gradually given up trying to keep up with him. They usually excused themselves by saying they were too busy. So he had responded by doing even more, trying to be even more available, to cover what wasn't getting done. He even confessed to becoming quite angry with some of his parishioners, questioning their faith, their personal motivation, and where their loyalties lay. I encouraged him to spend some time reflecting on others' negative attitudes and behaviours, but only after I had shared my recognition of how, understandably, he felt hurt, disappointed, and even somewhat disillusioned.

To further understand where his feelings about people fitted into the bigger life perspective, we then talked about his home life. He finally admitted that even there, his usual contented way of being the generous nice guy was fast disappearing. He noted in fact that he was sick of doing the extra chores that he now saw others could well have been contributing as their fair share. He was even contemplating bailing out of his marriage. His two small children were often sick, and the house seemed always to be in a mess. He felt tired and resentful of just being taken for granted.

On further reflection with him, he agreed that this feeling of being used had been there for a very long time, even within his family of origin. His emotional reactions to life in general, as expressed to me, indicated a deep feeling of despair. But now, at least he was beginning to self-reflect more honestly, clearly appreciating this opportunity and time to vent, without any fear of judgement or criticism.

I hope you can appreciate why it is always important in such situations to push for more details, even though this may be disturbing for the person and also for you as the carer/helper. In this example, when James was asked how seriously he thought about getting away from it all, he responded almost inaudibly. He admitted he had considered driving into a truck on several occasions, but something always held him back. Serious stuff – that just can't be left hanging. Further follow-on questions were needed: asking how he felt immediately before such thoughts, and also immediately afterwards.

Remember: feelings can mask the real issues.

Some time had passed since that wake-up call and, as expected, it had finally convinced the pastor helper that *he* needed to seek help. Here with me, in a safe place to speak openly, he was asked how he now felt about not having acted on his feelings at the time. More honest emotions were then admitted to. When I asked how he would cope if that impulsive reaction had left him with serious injuries, his response of an apologetic laugh provided me with some relief. Getting someone to the point of a reality check about the implications of such a catastrophic action can be a first step in helping a person to honestly start to identify the real issues needing to be faced.

After his almost 30 years of vocational service, it was important for me to affirm this man's present feelings of not being appreciated: James firstly needed to know that many others felt the same way. It was also important that he identified where he was at: feeling hopeless and overwhelmed. He also needed an affirmation of *my* understanding, of the unremitting impact of his constant grappling with the demands of others, with an enduring desire to be always available, yet seeing no end in sight.

A personal interchange about the advice he might give to someone else in his position proved to be quite important. You see, now that his emotional responses to his circumstances had been aired and understood, his ability to see things more rationally came to the fore. At this point it was unnecessary for me to provide such insights: James could now grasp for himself what alternatives might at least need to be considered. This of course confirmed a positive belief that, theoretically at least, he had always maintained: we all have choices. While his hidden and unexpressed *feelings* overwhelmed his thinking, thinking reasonably and rationally was often not possible.

Recall again from Chapter 3 – reflecting feelings *first* leads to greater understanding.

It is also relevant that we understand the importance of being able to teach the need to use assertive rather than permissive language, particularly when overcoming barriers to unacceptable behavioural patterns that need to change. You may need to refresh your memory by revisiting Chapter 2, under "Submissive, aggressive versus assertive communications".

Homework is great for self-reflection

After such an interchange, time alone is always needed for honest reflection, with follow-up thinking ensuring that decisions made are personally confirmed by an action plan. If James was to believe *he* owned this problem, rather than that someone else was responsible for making him feel bad, reflective homework was essential, to enable him to take personal responsibility for making liberating changes possible.

James was tasked with putting his newly formed conclusions about such alternatives in writing, ready for engaging in his next session about best options. In this instance, he was encouraged to take responsibility for posting up and constantly reviewing the oft-quoted Serenity Prayer of Niebuhr (1982–1971):

> *"God grant me the serenity to*
> *accept the things I cannot change,*
> *courage to change the things I can,*
> *and wisdom to know the difference."*

In James's case we again see, no matter how cognitively oriented and reasonable a person seems, the essential importance of sharing feelings *before* even considering imperative and rational alternatives. Remind yourself of characters in earlier chapters, like Sam (Chapter 2) and Martha's family of adult children (Chapter 3). It is sometimes helpful to consider feelings as being like a fog or smog that descends, occluding the light of day that normally reveals what is really there. While the smog remains, life seems dark and depressing, making it impossible to get a clear picture of the problem, to see what needs to change, let alone know how to achieve these potentially freeing lifestyle transformations.

Problem ownership – whose is the problem?

If we can go back to the idea of problem ownership,[1] as suggested in James's case, we see a man who felt helpless, believing the blame for his situation lay at the feet of others, until he realised for himself that the problem was indeed his to own. To gain the needed sense of ownership, he needed to come to himself, to his own realisation, not to be told what he should do, nor just have it explained. Perhaps this is now a good time to look at other situations which clarify what we really mean when we ask: who owns the problem?

Here is a behaviour diagram that might help:

BEHAVIOUR WINDOW		
Behaviour	*Problem ownership*	*What do I need?*
Acceptable Behaviour	Other person has a problem I have no problem	Helping and support skills: Active listening and respect
	No-one has a problem	Normal Relationship
Unacceptable Behaviour	I have a problem Other person - no problem	Assertiveness Skills: Respectful "I-message(s)"
	We both have a problem which we agree to own	Conflict resolution skills: collaboration, negotiation, win-win

Figure 4.1 Behaviour window

Let's think about a teenager who refuses to keep her room tidy, claiming it doesn't bother her. Is it a problem for her? It seems not. But her parent keeps bringing it up, with increasing frustration for both parent and child. This results in a continual conflict that flows into other areas of life – non-cooperation with routine tasks like breakfast times or completing homework, getting to school on time or procrastination with agreed domestic jobs – meaning that almost every interchange becomes a need for repetitive nagging. The relationship breakdown seems to have no easy solution.

Consider more specifically such a complaint about teenager Suzie, whose parent Joan initially thinks she has a right to be angry at her child for not keeping her room tidy, believing that Suzie is the problem. Joan reports being frustrated and feels really disturbed by Suzie's lack of thinking about the needs of the rest of the family, putting it down to her being a selfish kid who should be punished! To resolve "the problem" Joan needs to understand that the problem is actually hers to own: as far as Suzie is concerned, there isn't a problem. She believes that her mother is just wanting control! Feeling resentful of control by her mother (not the untidy room or her behaviour) is Suzie's problem, if she were to own a problem. So Joan judges Suzie to be selfish, and Suzie judges her mum to be controlling.

When Joan identifies and begins to understand that it is she who finds Suzie's behaviour unacceptable, she can then begin to resolve it; but only when she accepts that the problem to be solved is really her responsibility. Remember the point: the problem is not Suzie's, since she does not admit to having a problem with her untidy room. However, she does need to know that her Mum has a problem, namely with her own negative feelings as a consequence of her daughter's behaviour.

I-statements versus You-statements

The solution: in Joan deciding to engage Suzie the teenager in a non-threatening, non-emotional discussion, she needs to let Suzie know how her behaviour has become a problem for her as a mother. Such a discussion needs to take place when an appropriate, peaceable time is available, without any over-the-top negative emotions that could spoil the interchange. It should follow this sort of format:

Joan: Suzie, I have a real problem that I need your help with. Can we discuss this together?

[This is called an "I-statement" and compares with the normal "You-statement" which is accusative, and naturally brings out an angry defensive retaliation.]

Suzie: Sure, Mum, what's up?

Joan: Well, I understand that my reaction to you not keeping your room tidy is an issue for me, which is obviously not a problem for you, so *I* need to do something about that. You probably feel pretty angry with me always being on your back. Am I right?

Suzie: Yeah, that's right, cos I don't see it's any of your business how I keep my room! I usually keep my door shut!!

Joan: Yes, you do, Suzie. I appreciate that. And I'm sorry I've been on your back all the time. But where I have a problem is when I finish up having to take you to school because you've missed the bus. I know it's frustrating for you because you can't find something, like your school uniform, or your bag, then you get too late for breakfast . . . but then, because I have to take you to school, that mucks up *my* morning plans, makes me feel really frustrated, even angry and resentful. I then feel like my needs are irrelevant.

You can see Joan's statement here of her problem: this is the time when an assertive, but non-threatening I-message can potentially bring about a resolution. It doesn't try to downplay how one feels, but it does involve using the best alternative to the commonly used aggressive or permissive messages which you may remember we briefly referred to early in Chapter 1 and more fully in Chapter 2.

The most effective I-message involves a deliberate three-part statement:

1. <u>The problem</u>, identified with an I-statement – in this case an untidy room (that frequently means Suzie can't find whatever she needs), so Joan is needed to take her to school.
2. <u>The implications</u> or effects of the problem: here it can be identified as the effects on both Suzie (through loss of time, which means she misses breakfast and is too late to catch the bus) and more particularly on her mother (because taking Suzie to school disrupts her plans for the day).
3. <u>The feelings</u> are clearly declared – Joan really feels annoyed, resentful about being taken for granted by her daughter. You can imagine that even without spelling them out, there will likely be additional impacts on others in the family, as Joan's problem regularly becomes apparent to all!

When the relationship is respectful and caring, such a discussion can achieve great cooperation, particularly when there's a willingness by both parties to want to resolve the problem. Often this is evidenced by a child's response of "I'm sorry Mum but . . .". However, this is not always the case. The recipient of news of their unacceptable behaviour, even given in the best way possible by a caring I-statement, can still elicit quite a strong retort. This then requires the listener to be able to maintain a non-judgemental approach, making reflective statements about the <u>*other's feelings.*</u>

Such an interchange, after a considered, thoughtful three-way statement of the problem given above, might sound like this:

Joan: So you feel I shouldn't be upset or be frustrated by your untidy room, which because that means you can't find clothes I then have to interrupt my day to take you to school?

Suzie: I've told you, I can usually find my own stuff, and it doesn't matter to me if I miss breakfast, and I don't care if I'm late for school!

Joan (calmly, reflecting on the child's response): So you think it's unfair of me to bring this up as a problem, because you are not always late – so you feel I should just get over it, yeah?

Suzie: Yes, you sound like I am always late, which I'm not!

Joan: And you wish I could just ignore the many times when my day is mucked around because I need to drive you to school . . .

Suzie: Well, it doesn't happen that often does it?

Joan: From your perspective, you feel like it is not a big deal.

Suzie: That's right, no big deal really.

Joan continues (reiterating the problem issue with another I-statement): I can understand that from your perspective, Suzie. But since it happens often enough to be a problem for me that I frequently feel upset, I do think we should together try to find a solution to uniforms being lost, of you being short of time so missing the bus, and me having to drive you. I can't fix this problem or my reactive feelings without your help!

Suzie: Well, I admit I'm not the tidiest person, and sometimes clothes get on top of me when I don't get to putting them away . . .

Joan: So you do feel frustrated too, yeah? (Child nods.) So is there something I could do to help you be a bit more organised? Or maybe, do we need to find more shelves for your room? Or maybe you have other suggestions so that I don't keep being a frustrated, nagging mum!

> *Feelings really listened to leads to reduced reactions when linked with I-statements*

Can you see that when a problem is owned, *and* without using blame language, a mutually respectful discussion about alternatives makes resolving the problem more possible? Sharing the problem gains cooperation in finding mutually satisfying solutions! It clearly asserts the problem, shares feelings honestly, takes ownership of that problem, but engages the other in the finding of a solution.

This mirroring or reflection of feelings is the key response to an interchange where there are strong feelings expressed. This requires a *change in gears*[2] – from stating the problem (three-part), followed by listening to the reactive feelings of the other. You can imagine that the more strongly worded responses will need several minutes of simply staying with the feelings expressed, before *reiterating* the well-formed carefully worded I-statement given at the initial confrontation. This will mean that the person who has the problem needs to be willing and able to speak about the problem without overemphasising the emotions it causes them.

Whether the strong feelings are expressed within normal family exchanges, or coming from a person unhappy about the curved-ball circumstances life seems to have thrown at them, the mirroring of feelings is like saying "I can see that really has upset/hurt/made you feel useless . . ." and is a wonderful and powerful way to show you understand and have really heard.

However, too often people resort to saying inappropriate things like: "Yeah, I know how you feel . . ." And as already mentioned, the hurting person may rightfully be thinking: "you can't *possibly* know how I feel" – which means that your best intention to affirm where the person is at fails dismally. Acknowledging that you want to understand from them *how* they are feeling simply means asking "Does that make you feel . . .?". This is not ever going to be a problem, even if you get it wrong, because it is just that, a question. So the feeling experienced can then be clarified, and a better understanding agreed upon, building a greater likelihood of a more trusted relationship. Remember the interchange from Chapter 1 between the run-away boy Tom and me: trying to suggest you understand by asking a rhetorical question but getting it wrong is not a failure!

Owning the problem means that we admit to something as being an issue for us personally, and this becomes easy to understand when we recognise that such an issue does not bother the other person. Bringing this to the awareness of the other, however, is only going to create a war if we resort to blame statements that might typically be found in a finger-pointing angry You-message: "You are such a . . . because you always . . . and you don't care about . . ." All such attempts to get cooperation in solving a problem will meet with huge resentment, stubborn silence, and consequent non-resolutions.

Clearly, we can agree that a problem which involves another needs the assistance of the other, but once we accept *ownership* of that problem, expressed with an I-message, we will noticeably reduce the reaction that would result from a You-message. It does not necessarily eliminate it completely, however. After all, none of us likes to be pulled up, even when it is done gently.

Let's imagine, for example, that you had a habit of always leaving the table for me to clear away – perhaps innocently assuming that task was not your responsibility. I, however, who always do the clean-up, finally gets tired of it – so what do you think my eventual reaction might be? Probably anger, making a petulant outburst with: "you always leave me to clear the table and that's not fair!" Owning the problem does involve identifying and sharing your feelings, but without the accusations.

Alternatively, if in giving an I-message the frustrated me says: "I really feel resentful that when we've finished eating, it seems like I'm always left to clean up, or it means the dining table is left a mess until it's time to eat again, which I really hate seeing. This also leaves me really feeling taken for granted." No hurtful blaming: just an honest personal statement about the problem, its impact, and how one is feeling. Can you imagine how *you* might feel differently with this second approach to solve a problem, as compared to the first? Yes, a childish response may still have you defending your own neglect, with some dismissive ideas being expressed. But in this scenario, I in stating the problem would then need to shift gears, actively to listen to *your* surprised, reactive feelings by saying: "So you think I should be happy to clean up after every meal? You feel I am criticising you unfairly?"

Now your response to that might wish to further adjust that problem concept, suggesting you'd thought I was happy with the pattern of always cleaning up, but still not want to be involved with a solution, until I listen to *your* more apparent defensive feelings, like your saying: "Gosh, aren't you stirred up today – didn't you sleep well? Get out of the wrong side of the bed, hey?" This would then necessitate my shifting gears again, to encourage more of your thoughts and feelings, saying, "So you feel annoyed about my bringing this up, as if it's a petty thing that doesn't deserve attention?"

Such a conversation, particularly if felt as a really big issue by the one expressing the I-message, might take a few minutes of back and forth, stating the original message, followed by changing gears to listening to the reactive feelings, followed again by the I-message, before finally agreeing on an acceptable resolution.

Try it out! Understand that the benefits far outweigh the discomfort of leaving things be. Again, remind yourself of Sam, who had wrongly believed that avoiding a problem was the only option (Chapter 2). Resolution through using an I-message, followed by active reflection of the other's feelings, then restating the I-message finally creates less friction and can bring about a harmonious resolution while actually growing the relationship. Regardless of mutual satisfaction with the changes achieved, at least the status quo that had one person feeling taken advantage of will have been successfully both challenged and halted.

When is it appropriate to use a You-message?

This is appropriate when there is no problem, and where the relationship is such that stating the obvious need will be understood in its context. An example is "please, just shut the door . . . wipe your feet . . ." Alternatively if you are too tired but still want to resolve the issue at a future time, you can use a You-message, implied by saying, "Sorry, just leave it for now – I'm not up to a discussion right now; let's resolve this better, say, in the morning, hey?"

It is also right to use a direct instruction when an emergency requires immediate action, and this will be willingly accepted and deemed appropriate if not overused: "Watch out . . . get off the road!"; "Stop! Look!"; "Turn down the TV/radio! I can't hear you!"

Using these less destructive alternate ways of problem solving does not mean they will ipso facto all be resolved. Just reflect once more on Sam, from Chapter 2, who finally understood the need to use these tools, both in declaring his problem of unmet needs in the workplace, and who also became skilled in applying good listening skills to the reactive feelings from his management. However, he was not ever going to get a completely satisfactory response from the management without a mutual intent for harmony. The workplace today is frequently driven by economic rationalism, with personal and relational satisfaction often deemed irrelevant. Resolving the problem became his alone, because when a relationship is of no concern, joint ownership for problem resolution is rarely possible – unless of course a legal dispute sadly becomes necessary.

REVISION EXERCISES

- *Make* an opportunity to engage in a satisfactory interchange about a hypothetical problem with a colleague, partner, or caring other. Take opposing views that might express strong feelings. Practise, simply by verbally reflecting on or being a mirror to another's feelings, before moving on to confronting the next part of the argument or discussion. Experience what it is like to *feel* understood. Remember, the better the mirror, the more accurate your reflections are of the real issue. Don't forget to return to the original message that needs to be heard and acted on, hopefully with both in agreement.
- Reread this last chapter, particularly noting the clients reviewed, and try to write down as many questions as possible that you might have used to gain an understanding of the client's feelings. Then reflect on where this might have taken you next, in understanding the underlying issues.

Practice is needed to make mirroring of feelings become an automatic natural exchange in which you respond to unhappy information from others.

Otherwise, you will feel at sea in the interchange: potentially so overwhelmed by your own feelings that you are left confused about how to help the other.

- Revisit Chapter 1 and reflect on your empathic inclinations; check that these are healthy non-self-serving attitudes, rather than just compromising tools that make it difficult to create appropriate boundaries.
- The great Carer, always unselfish, encouraged us to love others *as we love ourselves*.
- How well do you practise this principle? This is not a selfish instruction, but a wise one that acknowledges we are limited humans; we need to take care of our own needs to avoid becoming empty, burnt-out vessels who have nothing left to give in the oft-draining care of others.

Remember: resolving a problem even with an I-message needs to be followed up with appropriate active listening before restatement of the problem.

Following your clear I-message (include the three parts), your active/reflective listening to the response is still usually required – return to genuinely listening to the other's reactive feelings, to reduce their negative feelings, before you reiterate the I-message.

Consider the following scenarios, then choose to carefully write a three part I-message for each, as opposed to the usual You-message you might have more easily framed!

Example 1. Your flatmate/partner regularly comes home late, insists on having a shower, and then plays music that you can't sleep through.

Identify

- The problem:
- The effects or implications on you:
- Your feelings:
- The I-statement:

Imagine the sort of feelings you may still have thrown back at you, to which you will effectively and actively listen, mirroring the other's responses/feelings, before then reiterating the I-message.

Example 2. Parents won't give you a house key, though you, an adult, drive your own car and hate the fact that they wait up for you to return home before going to bed themselves.

- Problem? Effects? Feelings?
- I-statement:
- Potential feelings you need to listen to:

Example 3. Boss at work treats you as an underdog, shows a lack of respect for your integrity, and takes for granted (rather than negotiating) your staying after hours.

Problem? Effects? Feelings? Now the I-statement. But remember, you will now need to reflectively listen! Then deliver your I-message again, for a resolution you can both agree to.

Notes

1 This empowering concept was originally developed by Dr Thomas Gordon in his various Effective Communication training programs. An internet search for <Problem Ownership Gordon> will yield a plethora of useful explanatory resources, videos and diagrams.

2 Look up the web on Effective Listening, also known as Active Listening, promoted by renowned psychologists Carl Rogers and Thomas Gordon.

Chapter 5

Strategies for dealing with emotional responses

This section of the book deals with many specific psychological issues that we as caregivers, professional or otherwise, need to be aware of. Here we focus on a variety of different skills needed to deal with issues often simply thought of as emotional problems. However, their associated habitual behaviours, exemplified by ineffective or destructive communications, or repetitive reactions, all suggest a need to question the inevitability of past behaviours controlling future behaviours. Such negative responses can potentially grow, for example, into a generalised anxiety, or an obsessive compulsive disorder, unless understood and appropriately confronted.

Relaxation is one effective counteraction, enabling opposing emotional responses to be resolved, and unconscious motivations brought into consciousness. Reflection again involves asking the right questions, ones that can identify what drives the response, and need to include what happened, how and when it happened, in order to expose and minimise any cumulative and diverse effects of trauma like grief and loss.

Good listening to others is an essential cornerstone for all interpersonal relationships, not just therapeutic ones. But listening is not just an interpersonal skill. We also need to understand the importance of regularly taking time out for ourselves, to reflect, and in that, the need to *listen to ourselves*, even more so when we are dealing with emotional concerns. At their core, all behaviours, both those that are good and those not so good, are shaped by thoughts and beliefs inside our heads.[1] We are often informed by our habituated and mostly unconscious self-talk. For example, when we blurt out our negative frustrations towards someone we usually treat well, what are we really believing about ourselves?

Perhaps "I deserve better than that", or even "I would never do/say what they just said". Though such inner attitudes or beliefs subconsciously control us, they may not really be the truth. If we really listen to and reflect on what we say and do, we may find there are some hidden beliefs that need to be reassessed, not simply excused. But as was already pointed out in Chapter 1, listening to oneself can be quite confronting, even difficult, but is essential if we are to better

DOI: 10.4324/9781003474746-5

understand ourselves and our sometimes less-mature behaviours! In that light, it is noteworthy that there is a reported increased interest in reflective journalling, leading to Apple Inc's release of an app intrinsic to their iPhone operating system.

The power of self-talk

As a small child, I often suffered from asthmatic attacks that were brought on by anxiety, though of course at the time I did not understand that. Frequent enforced rests meant I had many opportunities to think reflectively about my home life, where some parental patterns of behaviour left me sensing something was NQR (not quite right) in their impact on a whole family of individuals. In my later teen years, I became more able to identify some of these disturbing negative patterns. More importantly, this caused me to consciously decide which of these patterns I would *not* choose to follow. Yet I also became increasingly aware of some personal negative self-talk that still perpetuated, even though it was clearly unhelpful. The need to consider *alternatives* became a necessary part of my observations. Watching, learning, asking: how did *other* people live? What created harmony for them? What made *their* relationships work – maybe I could model on them?

When did *you* last reflect on how you behaved in a particular situation? Did you later wonder why that behaviour had occurred? I still find this necessary, even challenging old behaviours I had thought were gone forever! Taking time to reflect will often allow us opportunities to resist an old *reactive* behaviour before it happens again, and to think about appropriate ones that could considerably change future interchanges.

A brief aside: Behavioural change often requires more than just self-talk. Important adjuncts to changing behaviour are experiential. The use of Gestalt processes, of running through an imagination of behaving differently or role-playing an alternative, will be described in relation to changing habitual and addictive behaviours in Chapter 11.

Let's again think about what occurred with one interchange mentioned in Chapter 4, between the mother and teenage child. Joan had to rethink her past "normal" pattern of nagging then getting angry, trying to get Suzie to change her untidy room habit. There was nothing wrong with her goal, but she had obviously not thought about why her method was ineffective. Remember, the problem was really hers, not her daughter's.

One relevant and empowering question in such situations is to ask: "Can you remember someone in your life who used to do to or for you what you are now doing? Or, alternatively, you may have observed that same nagging directed towards one of your siblings, or maybe one parent to the other?" The answer, drawn out by asking and waiting for the person to carefully reflect on the past, creates a wonderful possibility for recognising the source of the pattern that allowed this problem to remain so long. This is also the case when a person says things like "I can't help myself". This underlying belief can equally apply to worthy behaviours, such as always seeking to make others feel better, like James had done for too long (Chapter 4). But such *unconscious automatic* responses may often drive the person, rather than be consciously selected behaviours that may be more appropriate.

Past behaviour need not remain the best predictor of future behaviour – a statement relevant to consider even when there are serious pathological issues.

One couple who came for relationship counselling had never really thought about what had contributed to their antagonistic way of relating to each other. Their genuine fears about eventually having to separate caused them to finally face a potential future apart. Very real anxieties expressed by both, particularly when visualising their single futures, raised many questions about how they would cope. Such concerns were obviously compounded by their fears of what an impact of their decision to separate would have on their children. Such a fear, disturbingly felt even in the midst of their antagonistic exchanges, at least gave them a common goal: to know how to protect their children from what they imagined as potential fearful consequences of a seemingly inevitable separation. Rather than expecting to achieve harmony within their own relationship, however, they obviously came seeking help that would at best minimise the impact of separation on their children.

Both parents were asked about their individual and respectively hurtful ways of communicating. After all, once separated, they agreed they would still need to communicate with kindness and consideration, at least when their children were present! I wondered with them about who had shown them such destructive ways of treating the person they loved. Cheryl, a forty-year-old, said with a look of surprise on her face: "I'd always said I'd never be like my Mum, but I'm doing just that!" Likewise, the husband eventually revealed that his aggressive way of putting her down, particularly in front of the kids, was very like the father he had come to hate – to the extent that as a young adult, Graham had determined never to see him again.

Self-fulfilling prophecy – unconsciously adopted

How often are such reflections on the past shared! In these instances people are then faced with a somewhat daunting challenge: the need to discard an old unrecognised pattern of their modelled behaviour and then, more importantly, to adopt a new one. Graham and Cheryl had not realised that their very anxieties carried from the past had been adopted as part of their own way of behaving towards their important other. The challenge was to see such attitudes and behaviours that were modelled to them should not carry on to yet another generation.

Part of the challenge for this couple was to start reflecting on alternative ways that they would *like* the other to speak to them. These needed to be reflected on singly, before articulating that to the other, and without any consideration of the *likelihood* that this might even be possible! This homework was then brought back to the next session, where together we could begin to explore how they could be helped to make such radical changes effectively.

More about relationships will be explored in Chapters 11 and 12. But for now, this couple had to face their anxieties, and to realistically grasp the changes that needed to be made to their current communication styles. Listening was not enough, so learning some new strategies became an essential ingredient, to potentially enable a more positive future. At the same time, this process effectively was able to remove their apprehensions, created by the inappropriate past that still distressed and controlled their respectively dysfunctional behaviours. Again, role-playing, along with healthy laughing at their past foibles, formed an important part of helping them adopt constructive alternatives. It was so good to see how a new perspective on their past provided a way to seeing and grasping a new future, and without needing to separate!

It is interesting that fear can also be a great motivator, even daring this couple to seek help to make changes – recognition that if this pattern had continued, the imagined fears could well have developed into full-blown anxieties, taken on by any one of the family members. You may even have wondered if this anxiety was simply an inherited problem: "What can you expect? Her father was a very anxious person!" Such anxiety is frequently exhibited by behavioural disturbances. These are more frequently observed with children than with adults, but as seen here are equally persistent and physically debilitating. But in this current example, their fears were identified and faced, and consequential anxiety as a long-term mental health problem avoided.

While this couple came concerned about how problems arising from their separation might impact their children, their issue was not one of wanting to work to stay together. They came to realise that the drivers for separation would not only impact them but would continue to be a problem for the children. Dealing with these as inherited relational patterns changed even their desire to separate.

Strong reactions emerge in many forms

We need to return briefly to James, the pastor (first mentioned in Chapter 4) who loved helping people but who could never draw a boundary line. His pattern of behaviour warranted a great deal of personal reflection: to carefully analyse his persistent need to be liked which drove most of his actions. Was this something that had been modelled to him, or was it something he had taken on for himself, as a way of dealing with family issues? And why did he believe he needed to take on so much responsibility for others?

Initial understanding came to him when he realised the impact of his own fear of failure: this had impacted his very worthy desire to encourage *others* to be equally responsible. This had proved too demanding, however, which had left him feeling he should simply retreat to holding only himself responsible, and for everything! Eventually, James needed to permit himself greater freedom to just be himself, rather than trying to live up to either his *Ideal* Self, or the expectations of others, the *Expected* self he mostly adhered to. More of this in Chapter 14.

Suffice it is to say here, James's fear of rejection by others had largely contributed to a life where burnout formed a cyclic pattern. We see a man driven by an inability or refusal to rethink his early commitment to needing to be liked, along with his failure to say no assertively. At times his fears became so demanding that physiological reactions to stress such as his high blood pressure, and concomitant psychological anxieties about his health, had led to frequent withdrawals from work. James had not developed legitimate ways to create, let alone action, a work/life balance. The balance had never been consciously considered or thought possible.

As we reflect on the examples of the people I was privileged to work with, it will be clear that self-reflections generate a need for different approaches. Let's reflect on Thomas, a 67-year-old man who needed to have an MRI before a major hand operation. He had flatly refused to go ahead with what for him was proving to be an anxiety-ridden task, hence the referral to a psychologist. Thomas unwillingly attended his first session, exhibiting a great deal of anxiety. The consulting room being quite small, he said he felt claustrophobic. Maybe this suggested agoraphobia, I hear you say? Maybe PTSD and, if so, why? He refused to sit down so I needed to find a suitable alternative location where he could share his serious medical problem. His dilemma? Either to accept a fast-deteriorating ability to use his hand, or to access possible medical knowledge and treatment that would prevent this. But this was only possible if he would face whatever had started his present anxiety.

A public lake was nearby, so he agreed to take a walk out in the fresh air. During that time outside, followed by time sitting in quiet contemplation, Thomas was more able to reflect on his recently identified anxiety. He had not previously wondered about *why* he had such a debilitating reaction. Those important questions again: asking him to go back to a time when he remembered first feeling anxious. After finally feeling quite relaxed, he recalled his first feelings of being stifled, remembering having been incarcerated, way back as a small child under a rubble of concrete, after a bomb had hit and demolished his home during

World War 2. He was found two days later. Though this event had not remained a *conscious* trauma for the many years since, more recent media coverage of a similarly traumatic incident had suddenly startled him into a deep awareness of the fragility of life. That event had been reported in detail, with the media reporting the trauma experienced by a man caught and buried in the snow during an avalanche in the Victorian Alps.

Further questioning of past situations revealed that Thomas had experienced several quite amazing near-tragedies, but each time he had simply been able to put it aside and, successfully he said, had "just got on with living". He had never thought of himself as an anxious person. But now these traumas all seemed to have caught up with him.

Being now required to enter a very confining tunnel to deal with his latest medical problem had suddenly caused him to feel overwhelmed. His present severe reaction illustrates what can be called the last-straw effect. This is observed when there is a cumulative effect of a variety of life experiences that, though largely unconscious and untroubling, had indeed been quite traumatic in themselves. His presentation now suggested that he was suffering from a resulting generalised anxiety problem.

Generalised anxiety – using relaxation, one step at a time

The second session was sitting again beside the lake, the setting incorporated into effectively teaching him to relax. While there, a traumatic event that came to mind was one which clearly had been treated as trivial at the time, but now resurfaced as part of the accumulated stressors. While he was sleeping in his caravan, a flooded dam higher up the hill had burst, washing him and his van into the nearby lake. He could now even recall this with some laughter! Now beside another lake, Thomas learnt to comfortably close his eyes, to simply imagine seeing the water, the trees, and the people travelling nearby. It involved him learning how to tense up every muscle he could and then to release these, appreciating a sense of calm, being relaxed.

Experiencing relaxation in a safe place enabled Thomas to remember some of the difficult situations he had successfully lived through. While being relaxed, he could now begin to see these situations without experiencing the same involuntary *visceral* body reactions previously felt in relation to the perceived threat of an MRI (the visceral response being an autonomic body reaction, not consciously mediated). The lessening body reactions, achieved by using systematic desensitisation to visualise the past events while concomitantly relaxed, helped Thomas feel some relief, and start to believe in his potential ability to face his next hurdle.

Perhaps you need to check out the reality of some personal visceral responses that get *your* heart racing, so just now reflect on those things that involuntarily make your sweat glands embarrass you. How do you manage them? On what are those anxious reactions based? Having applied this approach to your own perceptions, what do you think would best help Thomas at this stage of his self-awareness?

Though generalised anxiety can be more difficult to overcome, we can consider it essentially like climbing a mountain – step by step, one hurdle after another, breaking down the complexities into manageable bite sizes for desensitisation. Often it is important to identify a common thread, though each fear/anxious belief may need to be attended to in relation to specific memories that have contributed to identified current fears or threats. Part of this review process with Thomas would hold the positive key benefit, of what he'd experienced as resilience in the past might now be reclaimed, a strength not previously acknowledged.

As relaxation effectively countered his anxiety, the various traumatic experiences Thomas had lived through in greater detail were exposed, and his clear and wondrous ability to have endured these without too much long-term distress was revealed. The next step for Thomas was to attend his third and fourth relaxation sessions in the consulting room, during which he was introduced to his strongest irrational fear. This was enabled by his simply watching an imaginary TV screen, instructed to observe other individuals undergo an MRI in a hospital. Using this method of confronting fearful situations is a powerful means by which a person can more easily disassociate the painful scenario from the personal experience, watching it from a safe distance. This then became another step towards imagining *himself* being in the theatre, and eventually relaxed, to imagining himself moving into the MRI tunnel: a form of Systematic Desensitisation.[2]

You can see that this gradual process involved not only visualising a number of past events from which he had amazingly survived, but also involved developing more confidence. As he verbalised his feelings about these, he could then recognise his current situation as being far less fear-inducing.

Realistically and rationally evaluating the small likelihood of the MRI being a traumatic event then became part of his more cognitive therapy. Together these techniques allowed Thomas to again grasp the positive elements from his past lived experiences, reflect on his incredible earlier facility to handle and overcome the many difficulties of his past, and to apply this newly conscious self-confidence to the upcoming new experience. He was also encouraged to choose a particular piece of music that he enjoyed, and to utilise this comfort at home while regularly repeating relaxation exercises. He appreciated how important this would be for him within the imaging chamber. It was no longer considered an underground chamber of horrors but reframed to him experientially: as a great potential for bringing about healing while listening to music.

Noteworthy about this approach is its gentleness and holistic comprehensiveness. Together we did not simply focus on his presenting problem but saw it as the last straw in a *series* of events. The other memories were considered equally significant in terms of needing to be addressed to minimise a future need for help, but only if or when those stressors arose.

Relaxation – imagery formed from personal experiences

When employing a formal use of relaxation,[3] it is important that we find what really relates to the life experiences of the person seeking to change an unacceptable reactive behaviour. Remember to check what sort of things may relax the person, rather than assuming you know what will relax them. Some will tell you they relax with quiet, bush scenes, while others relax in a bustling shopping centre or riding on the back of a fast-moving motor bike! I remember engaging with a tense, overanxious lady in a closed-eyes relaxation experience that I thought she would enjoy. Mid-way through my exploring a simple muscle-relaxing episode, followed by audibly painting a beautiful scene for her, Helena suddenly opened her eyes and said: "Actually, I am in the snow, up on a mountain, not down on the beach!" Though the *faux pas* was overcome with laughter, uncovering that information first before commencing a relaxation episode had been a missed opportunity, and obviously applies equally to any person who expresses a phobia – of spiders, say, or of going to the dentist.

Can you think what other questions you would ask people about each of such potentially fearful situations, before creating a relaxation programme?

Remember to ask What, When, How, or Where questions,
but ***not*** *Why!!*

Asking "why" belongs to rational discussions, not in those interactions and situations where emotions may run high or deep. Recall Joan and Suzie (Chapter 4), and note the confounding effect that emotions can have. The "why" question may only provide a rational response that is very little other than an excuse or feeling, but not be the real reason!

Perhaps we can now focus on what sort of events or demands make *you* feel anxious. How do you manage them? Do you effectively use positive self-talk, saying things like "I know this can be quite stressful, but I know I've managed it before so I'll just ignore this"? Perhaps you try to do something which takes your mind off the anxiety created, not allowing yourself the time to explore your feelings, because these are thought at best to be irrelevant, trivial, childish, just needing to be buried, or deliberately repressed.

This last option can work well for a time, as it had for Thomas. But in the end, our feelings can be triggered by something unexpected, and then surprisingly get the upper hand, demanding they are heard – which clearly suggests that they *are* important.

One of the many people of differing ages and situations needing help to overcome a variety of debilitating anxieties comes to mind. Kylie had been an "ambo" (common Australian term for paramedic) for some years, and she reported loving her work. But for three months since her last callout, she had found she couldn't face going to work. She was angry at herself for becoming what she regarded as "so pathetic". After all, she said her last retrieval had not been a big deal, as she had seen many such bad accidents in the past. In fact, she said, some were even worse.

Our natural reaction for someone so experienced is to wonder: *why* this sudden reaction now? But questioning *how* this last accident might have been different from previous events allowed her to recall one small detail that was indeed different: the child she had rescued from a burning car was only three years old. Kylie remembered registering at the time that her own youngest child, with the same blond hair, was only one year older.

When self-talk is not enough

Her usual self-talk about how she had coped with such traumas before, and "now she was just being ridiculous" was not working; neither was her refusal to sit still long enough, simply to avoid thinking about her own feelings. She reported getting up early before work to go running, which in the past had always done the trick in coping with any reticence to go to work, but now, getting to work remained impossible.

Kylie was surprised that, in her own words, her body seemed to have taken over her life, with uninvited visceral hot sweats, feeling physically nauseous whenever thinking about work, lying awake at night, worrying about anything and everything, making sleep impossible. Overtiredness then took on another form: eating became a new way of temporarily helping her feel less anxious.

Before long, however, the anxious symptoms reappeared, along with beating herself up about her eating habits, comfort eating that meant she had put on a lot of unwelcome weight. Finally, her boss at work, having been to workshops on post-traumatic stress, had insisted on her attending the trauma counselling that previously she had always dismissed and seen as a sign of weakness.

For Kylie – as is the case with so many others in professions where they become well used to confronting disturbing accidents (or like that experienced by Thomas) – accumulated effects meant that this last final straw had broken through her capacity to deny and detach. On review, Kylie clearly had a mountain of traumas with no way out but to work through them. She admitted that at first this reaction had been a real hit to her pride – she had never needed help before, so why now?

Cumulative effect of trauma leading to anxiety

It was apparent to Kylie, after crying her way through her first session, that she needed to take time out, to deliberately reflect on her own vulnerability, as a person and as a parent; her own mortality and that of her children; and her own presumption that she would always be able to stay in control, and "on top of her feelings".

Healing for Kylie took several months, retelling much of her life's pattern of living with unexpressed traumas, now full of deeper reflections. Her earlier experiences evidenced some deeply buried experiences she had simply brushed away, but which ultimately were important to recall, learn from, and deal with. She recalled one event after another that might have reminded her of as yet unexpressed griefs – like losing her precious Dad at an early age, though for the most part she had deliberately refused to remember that time, desperately intent on keeping unhappy thoughts out of her conscious awareness.

Finally, her being able to share her grief in a safe place, and with someone who held no false expectations of her, was in and of itself a huge salve to her inner anxieties that until now had unwittingly begun to control her. As was remarked on earlier with Thomas, research shows how important it was that Kylie understood the well-established body of research on a post-traumatic response. This clearly testifies to the cumulative effect of many and often quite differently distressing experiences in ordinary, otherwise healthy individuals. It was important to help Kylie understand that her current reaction was not a sign of weakness or lack of self-control, but rather to be expected from anyone with normal healthy human awareness and sensitivities.

REFLECTIVE EXERCISES

- How well do you handle your own grief and loss? Spend some moments to catch the essence that sorrow or trauma has on your daily life. Consider their impact on your own ability to deal with situations you normally cope well with. With whom do you share your griefs?

Now transfer that understanding while thinking about how you manage other people's grief issues. Our response to others' grief may reflect our own expectations about how *we* personally deal with grief, in its various forms.

- Find ways of saying more than the formally accepted words of "I'm sorry for your loss". Regardless of how close we feel to the other, we certainly need to feel prepared to sincerely express our concern for their loss, with a more sympathetic understanding of what emotions they may need to share. Listen, then respond appropriately.

The next chapter places more focus on the various support methods that work best when we have an understanding of the underlying causes of how and why people *feel* so overwhelmed.

Notes

1 Questioning beliefs underlying self-talk is taken further in terms of adaptive and maladaptive schemas in Chapter 16.
2 For more detail look up "systematic desensitisation" on the internet. Especially relevant, https://en.wikipedia.org/wiki/Systematic_desensitization.
3 Look up various forms of alternate relaxation that consider body, mind, and spirit.

Chapter 6

Underlying issues require differing support options

By highlighting again the importance of feelings that control unwanted or undesirable behaviours, this chapter presents examples of clients who need to challenge what they believe about WHY their feelings exist. Often confronting such feelings means that the real problem is identified and relief given quite quickly, with long-term problems like PTSD avoided. Other times, secondary gain through emotional rationalisation provides a clarity that at least gives choices about future repercussions. Perceptions of experiences can benefit from being reviewed through a new perspective lens, like Seligman's 3 Ps, particularly when trusted carers can model alternative understandings to replace unhelpful old ones. Repetitious practice of such new understandings is demonstrably imperative for lasting change to be achieved.

Individual responses – when enough is enough

One example of how quickly anxious thinking can appear like a phobic reaction was seen in a small boy who was refusing to go to school. His mother June stated she felt at her wits' end, not knowing how to get young Max to school without a fight. He was eight, and until the last few months, had always loved going to school. June knew he was a sensitive, thoughtful boy, and she hated to see him distressed in any way. But he seemed unable to tell his mother why he didn't want to go to school, and this again clearly exemplifies how asking *why* will often get erroneous, irrational answers. Max kept giving his mother different reasons why he couldn't go to school: stomach ache; other times he said his knee hurt or his arm was sore and so on. He'd seen the doctor, who reassured June he could find no physical ailments – "probably just growing pains!" Maybe this answer meant, "I can't find any physical reason – perhaps there is something else going on that is of a more psychological nature?"

After getting Max to play with some Lego, and generally having him feel ok about being with me, I finally earned the right to go deeper with my questions. I asked him what days he would most likely to be unhappy at school, and he was clearly able to answer: Fridays.

DOI: 10.4324/9781003474746-6

He was then asked what happened on Fridays. Guess what? Yes, sport, something he really enjoyed. You'd be forgiven for thinking he didn't like reading and writing but only sport! More detailed questions, however, revealed that Mrs Green wasn't there on Fridays, so now there was a real Aha moment! Somehow, *she* was part of the problem. What questions did I need to ask now? Well yes, ones that sought to clarify what there was about this teacher that made Max not like school. Not *why*, but *what* did Mrs G do that he didn't like, that made him feel unhappy and afraid? "What" and "how" questions were given in simple words, asking Max to describe her unacceptable behaviour. These allowed him to answer specifically: she often spoke loudly, used unkind put-down words, and expected Max to jump quickly when she made demands.

His mother June now understood this to suggest that Mrs Green could be perceived as a bit of a bully. She had *felt* the teacher was not very patient with little boys, and agreed that she seemed to always have been particularly impatient with Max. On reflection, June realised herself that he could be quite slow in his thinking, and therefore was never fast in doing what he was told to do.

It was a relief to his mother to discover a reasonable explanation behind Max's non-attendance at school. She began to understand that his illness claims were what we call a rationalisation, giving an explanation that might mean he could avoid his pain. Here we have a cogent example of how the *why* question confounds issues. You will recognise how frequently even adults use the same technique when responding to the question "*why* did you do that?" in attempting to excuse/explain their behaviour that *should* have been reasonable rather than unacceptable! Sometimes these answers can even be quite convincing.

Counter rationalised explanations with competing relaxation and imagination.

The new challenge then entailed deciding what June should do about Mrs G – the mother's first and natural reaction was to look at changing schools. This session needed her to reflect with me alone, while young Max was happily ensconced in the waiting room with some toys. June was later encouraged to constructively talk with other parents about their own experience of the teacher. She discovered that she was not alone: some had already been to the school principal who informed them that the teacher was being counselled. Remaining at the school seemed a far better option than changing schools, because, with zoning in place, this move could only be to a non-government school; this was difficult, with cost, distance, and travel all inconvenient, and Max's friends were really important to him.

The teacher remained at the school, and some of her authoritarian impatience diminished, the teacher claiming simply to be "old school strict". It is interesting to note here, however, that once the problem was no longer concealed, and others had shared their concerns about the teacher, in subsequent sessions Max became more willing to think about what might make him feel better about the "bully" teacher: so building resilience was indicated. His imagination was called in, enabling him to recall cartoons of characters that showed how to treat bullies without either becoming a bully, or alternatively running away. He then imagined what he could do that would make him feel like laughing inside himself, even when the teacher made demands of him that were a bit scary. Max imagined her with a long Pinocchio nose, and he learned to "put this on her face" whenever he felt she was being mean. A more likely suggestion today might be to have a film-loving child describe his most disliked character in his favourite film. Max found this technique a powerful way of increasing his internal confidence, and as we role-played some scenarios together, he clearly demonstrated that he could effectively dismiss her unacceptable behaviour using this strategy.

The process of engaging Max in finding his own solution also helped his mother, because she was able to see that, ultimately, he only needed to be effectively listened to, and by including mirroring that clearly indicated she understood his feelings, a combined strategy created a way to effectively cope with his fears. In turn, she recognised that Max would learn to handle life, even potentially other bullies, with greater resilience than she'd done. June also recognised in herself a previous pattern of hiding from unkind people or running away when things seemed too difficult. Huge relief for both mother and child: a potential long-term school phobia was effectively dismissed before it could take hold.

Coping strategies

Developing skills that involve constructive internal coping strategies, such as Max learned, is so important. When used appropriately, these skills help the frustrated person avoid simply resorting to unnecessary confrontational interactions. Such negative engagement typically sets up a destructive culture of a victim-perpetrator yo-yo: where victims model on and learn to become perpetrators in order to win.

This last example in challenging patterns of difficult behaviour highlights some significant elements that make lasting new changes more possible. If for example I say, "don't think of the colour red", the natural response will automatically bring red to mind, yes? Unless of course you have either a compliant or defiant personality! In other words, when we decide to challenge a personal behaviour, we must first find a positive *alternative* that might achieve the required result. Think about Max: instead of focusing on Mrs G's hard, grimacing face, and unkind words, Max, with some necessary practice, became light-hearted when visualising her with a ridiculous long nose, thus creating a totally different internal feeling about her. The positive internal self-talk became part of his new response to her. School became a place where he could feel more in control, even with Mrs G. The old negative feeling of helpless victimisation and his new feelings were impossible to hold on to at the same time!

Relaxation: a competing positive response

In the case of Thomas, we have already pointed to an example of systematic desensitisation. In this technique you may already understand the powerful effect of relaxation paired with thinking about an anxiety-inducing behaviour or exposure. We see this for example in a phobia, such as with a fear of snakes, when completing anxiety-raising exams, or when learning to drive after an accident. Previous seemingly impossible behaviours can become possible when a person's imagination is explored while relaxed. Our minds can recall our imaginings as being as powerful as real memories. This form of virtual reality is commonly experienced, by children as well as adults.

I'm reminded of a lady we'll call Sabina whom I met after a referral from the Transport Accident Commission (TAC), a government insurance organisation that offered psychological as well as medical assistance after a serious car accident. She had spent some months in hospital, but now after many more months at home, she was deemed *physically* fit and expected to return to work. However, it was agreed that she needed some help in getting over the *psychological* effects of the accident, particularly as related to her lack of ability and confidence to drive to work. She expressed some difficulty even in being a passenger, and the thought of ever driving again seemed virtually impossible. I knew that controlled relaxation exercises would be essential if she was to regain any confidence in her ability to drive. Part of her therapy also involved a cognitive review of the likelihood of the same accident occurring again, and her sense of logic and her own rationality were clearly in her favour.

After the educative process, we worked through various situations, where a competing relaxed mode of thinking began to replace her relatively newly acquired feelings of anxiety about driving. Initially this involved Sabina simply being able to visualise herself sitting in the driver's seat while being relaxed. The next step involved her imagining seeing herself driving to the end of the road and back. A few sessions only were needed before she reported on her day-to-day lived experiences that demonstrated just how well she was doing, even allowing her partner to be her passenger, with him assisting only by being there. Sabina had then also thoughtfully commenced a defensive driving course, and these lessons she reported were going well. Her new positive thinking had clearly made a big impact in reducing her driving fears.

Surprisingly, some months later I received a phone call from her solicitor, asking if Sabina had recently returned for more therapy, and I wondered why he thought she needed more help. Soon after, another appointment was made by Sabina. She disclosed she had discontinued driving lessons, as she had been advised that her compensation from the accident would be seriously reduced if she was driving again! Secondary gain had risen its head: a side benefit received as a *dis*incentive to deal with a problem, though is not directly part of the issue needing attention. This now explained to me Sabina's decision to stay with her problem, so as not to risk the substantial potential financial downside of reduced compensation associated with moving on.

Here you might like to refresh your understanding of the powerful effect on how fast or how fully an individual may or may not regain health when secondary gain is present.

Secondary gain can prevent positive developments.

I had to accept an end to my role in Sabina's restored health, as the offer extended to her was too great to give up. I was disappointed for her, but sadly understood that, for the person seeking help, their healing will always be dependent on how seriously that person regards the worth of being well. It reminds me of the great Healer's question to the paralysed man, waiting for years by the healing waters for a cure: "do you really want to be well?" Sabina chose to stay "unwell" for the sake of a potential monetary benefit. I can only hope that down the track she made a new attempt to become whole. It is not unusual, however, that a stubborn deeply subconscious value, in this case financial benefits, along with other secondary gains have been known to hold a person back.

Feelings need to be expressed but are not meant to control.

Do you know what it feels like to be anxious? What do you initially tell yourself?

Remember how self-talk works, either to help or hinder you from becoming stuck. But when you appreciate that self-talk is often not as effective as you would like, then you need to become aware of potential next steps, for yourself as well as for others you may wish to help.

Suggested alternatives can provide positive inspiration for change. Sharing how *you* feel can help others not only identify those feelings, but also normalise their own reactions – for example, if they learn that being anxious in specific situations is commonly experienced. However, listening carefully to the additional concerns expressed can highlight underlying *patterns of thinking*.

Thoughts/cognitions that identify controlling beliefs

Being able to draw these out can enable one to challenge various wrong beliefs that have convinced the person they can't change. A feeling-based belief that the problem is *permanent* – "I will never get over it!" – can sometimes be contradicted if that belief is exaggerated, to the point that the sufferer sees the ridiculousness of maintaining that belief. Sometimes, though, this risks a greater problem for a more deeply entrenched negative thinker, requiring a next step.

This might include considering the ill-based belief as an *all-pervasive* conviction, that a particular anxiety will affect *everything*. Such thinking is often linked to another underlying and very *personal* negative belief. Ill-founded beliefs like these tend to involve people using exaggerated self-talk like "No one else ever feels like this", or "*Everyone* is out to get me", reminiscent of the pithy saying: "Nobody loves me, everybody hates me, I think I'll go and eat worms . . .!" Unfortunately, many who feel this way will choose a more palatable and addictive option: like eating more chocolate!

These three aspects of quite controlling negative beliefs demand a little more attention here.[1]

Seligman's 3 Ps for depression: Personal, Pervasive, Permanent

I remember one client who had become generally quite anxious, convinced about her inability to deal with any new demands. This *seemed* to have grown out of the mere thought of becoming pregnant, following some five years of marriage. That anxiety had extended into everyday activities, like worrying about cooking dinner, never being able to decide on what new clothes to buy for herself, and even being quite anxious about how they as a couple could ever afford to buy the new car they needed. These were just a few of the anxieties her husband shared with me, and about which, when they were aired, Mary clearly felt very embarrassed. They had an obvious commitment to each other, and Gerry's continuing patience with her anxieties was something she valued, though she feared this might soon run out.

What are your thoughts about this fearful lady? Where would your questions begin?

For a start, important data was needed: how long these fears had controlled her, how often they worried her, and when she thought the extreme range of anxieties had commenced. These were all valued questions, and Mary's anxieties were greatly clarified by having the insights of her loving husband. However, hearing her family of origin story over the next session or two, on her own, revealed some important elements that may have contributed to her present frame of mind. Mary had suffered much at the hands of an angry mother who had apparently suffered with undiagnosed mental health issues. This had also sadly resulted in Mary's father, the more confident quiet achiever, choosing to leave the family when she was only 12 years old. Mary came to admit the awful impact these family tragedies had had on her and her brother, leaving both seriously lacking the confidence and resilience required to deal with life's demands. She reported that her brother still lived alone, with continued great difficulty in making friends.

You may need to note that similar mental health issues experienced in a family have frequently been reported by the adult children, requiring greater understanding of the many elements that will demand attention, even years on. Do some further research if you really find this an important aspect of your caring for others.

In Mary's case, one of the more ongoing negative elements highlighted by her husband about her childhood was her mother's continual criticisms. She still insisted that Mary would "*never* be able to do . . ." a great string of things, and these had become powerful disincentives to her ever trying anything new or different. The fact that she had married was a great tribute to Gerry's loving persistence: he had seen her potential and had continued to encourage Mary to question many of her mother's abusive predictions against her that still held her captive.

Explore the past before changing the future

Some therapies – typically those with a psychodynamic orientation – advocate many sessions over a long period of time to explore past traumas. However, from a cognitive behavioural orientation, we find a careful questioning can reveal much that is important within a very short timeframe. For Mary, briefly exploring the depth of pain experienced throughout her childhood was an important part of her healing.

Relaxation exercises were also an important daily routine, and these became intertwined with imagining differences in her life. Being able to encourage her to reflect in writing about the many deceptions her mother had maintained became a way in which she could more easily disassociate from and clarify what specific beliefs needed to be discarded. The powerful method found manageable by Mary was for her to write out the beliefs she came to recognise as potential lies, and to check their veracity with either her brother or with Gerry before burning them. It was important that she also compose and write out *opposing* true statements, statements that effectively countered these false and irrational beliefs. These could then be highlighted and regularly referred to when in doubt.[2]

Asking Mary to deliberately reflect on any fears that might be good to retain was also essential – for example, appropriate concerns that would be necessary to protect her from harm. This encouraged her to discern the difference between making good thoughtful decisions and not being careful at all. It is well known that adult children of people with mental illness will need greater assistance in having a clear rationale for the choices they need to make. Clearly it becomes imperative that such people, impacted by dysfunctional relationships, need to know someone mentally stable they can safely relate to, thus providing a trustworthy relationship that is so important for their future well-being.

Strong safe relationships
encourage health-restoring self-beliefs and attitudes.

This aspect of Mary's own vulnerability created the need for her to be encouraged to think positively, and realistically, about how much she could trust Gerry's understanding of her. I too needed to gain a deeper understanding of Gerry and his own attitude to people and life's demands. Such knowledge was required to inform an essential assessment before accepting the efficacy of his role in her development, which ultimately contributed much to Mary becoming an independently healthy partner.

Confidence in this man's trustworthiness was therefore crucial before another step: encouraging her to consider ways in which she might unselfishly contribute to *Gerry's* needs, specifically in his desire to become a dad. It was exciting to see changes in her thinking when she no longer focused on her own negative beliefs. Her being more positive had included knowing herself more truthfully, so then she was more able to consider the significant other person in her life. She also began reading, giving herself permission to relax, learning to hear from others about how they managed new things. Along with growing self-confidence, gradually Mary extended her thinking to how a baby might contribute to their future happiness together.

When Mary shared how she felt about her mother's perspectives of her, then reconsidered herself in relation to Gerry, the efficacy of any potential changes powerfully took on a new positivity not felt in her early life. She could then more openly admit to her fears which became less dominant when she actually took responsibility for attempting new activities. For example, Mary had great fears about holding a baby, so being able to hold a friend's baby became one experience she reported as amazing and not nearly as difficult as she had expected. Imagining had to be tested alongside reality, and Gerry became her trusted and valued encourager.

Imagining – must relate to safe reality testing.

It was wonderfully heartening over the following year or more for me to occasionally see Mary's development, sharing her journey over the period of her pregnancy and eventual birth of a son. Of course there were times of doubt, when she needed to revisit the old, well-engrained negative self-beliefs (particularly when highlighted with the demands of new experiences), but my role was simply to take Mary back to newly formed beliefs about herself, reminding her that old irrational or untrue beliefs, like old habits, die hard. New habits and beliefs are often so much harder to become "the new normal", unless carefully and frequently reiterated and practised.

In reflecting on how you cope when anxious, you will surely notice the power of feelings, with various emotions that warrant attention. Remember, however, that unless those feelings are thoughtfully reconsidered, they will continue to speak into our lives, with an added complexity that can turn up the "noise" on the problem. Such confounding signals can make it difficult to hear the good and appropriate *new* alternate responses, meaning those *old* anxious, previously accepted subconscious irrational ideas can at vulnerable times still resurface, with times of stress becoming times of distress again.

In this chapter we have examined using relaxation in a process of dealing with cognitions associated with emotional stressors. Relaxation as a regular activity on its own, such as in mindfulness which involves diverting away from the cognitive, or as part of acceptance and commitment therapy, is worth further exploring. Good material is readily available in publications and on the internet.

REFLECTIVE EXERCISES

- Think of something that creates anxious reactions within yourself. Note how these affect your body. Check where you first remember them occurring. Write down your reflections.
- Then form alternate beliefs that fit well with your revised attitudes about life, including about who you trust, what knowledge backs up your beliefs, and what positive experiences you can lean on as *trustworthy*: all necessary answers that can inform your new attitudes, new beliefs.

Some of the examples of clients in earlier chapters may now have given you a greater insight into what may have contributed to their over-reactions. Many reactive behaviours had become part of the various individual behaviours that needed to be challenged, if not completely transformed. So revisit them now.

- Reread the boy Max's concerns with school with an open mind about how you would have questioned him, and perhaps how you might have responded to his feelings. You may have examples of other people you would like to help.
- Write up a potential plan, with some clear goals you might hope to achieve when sharing with them.

Note: in the same way that feelings can be overwhelming for the individual, it is important to consider the effects when a group of people share their experiences of anxieties. Wisdom is needed to both monitor and re-educate the group in how contagiously negativity can play out, especially when individual differences are not acknowledged. Even as we know that medication often has quite distinctly different side-effects on individuals, attention is also needed to consider uniquely personal reactions to experiences endured, as well as to therapeutic techniques and their efficacy for healing.

- Read up on Albert Ellis's 10 irrational beliefs, readily available in many books on Rational Emotional Behaviour Therapy (REBT), or online.[3]
- Explore further deeper understanding of irrational belief structures by digging into books on Jeffrey Young's Schema Therapy.[4]
- Consider the common *praxis* of the day, as compared with *phronesis*, which considers an *understanding* of why a particular practice needs re-evaluation in the light of experience that sheds light on the context in which it may or may not work. You may want to clarify phronesis as supporting an opinion that may not be commonly accepted but the wisdom of which cannot be denied.[5]

Be aware that some people respond quite quickly to new therapeutic insights, so that for them, it seems much like turning the page to a new chapter. For others, however, such changes are much more difficult to internalise – more like creating a new book from scratch! This latter individual needs the creative counsellor to be patient, to pace and lead, while also modelling the new preferred behaviour with a clear understanding about the individual's capacity or personal inclination to make changes. This will be given more attention in the later chapters as we refer to both abilities and different personality types.

We move on to the next chapter to deal with depression, a worldwide phenomenon suffered by more than 250 million people according to the World Health Organization (WHO) in January 2020. That was prior to the COVID19 pandemic! Before reading on, you may find it helpful to look up WHO definitions of anxiety disorders, as distinct from depressive disorders, as reported in their 2017 website.[6]

Notes

1 Consult the internet: Martin Seligman, Positive Psychology, the 3 Ps of resilience.
2 Look up Albert Ellis's 10 Irrational Beliefs where the core of a number of these and their rebuttal can be found as first-step alternatives.
3 Starting point: https://en.wikipedia.org/wiki/Rational_emotive_behavior_therapy.
4 Starting point: https://en.wikipedia.org/wiki/Schema_therapy.
5 Our hope in daring to write this book of our experiences (*praxis*) is that a clear understanding (*phronesis*) of what really works in caring for others may help you build confidence – though it must rest on truth, and on well validated theory that is tested for its efficacy and wisdom. These two Greek terms are widely applied to describing a reflective recursive process
6 An internet search on the terms "Depression Pandemic" will bring up the latest relevant World Health Organization pages as well as references to scholarly articles.

Chapter 7

Depression in various forms

Increasingly considered as a worldwide pandemic, depression is fleshed out in relation to cultural, personal, and circumstantial matters that are not always understood. Post-traumatic treatment options can be better discerned by knowing what exogenous (external) or endogenous (internal) elements may have combined to create lasting or repetitive episodes. Many factors may be potential contributors to depression, and the carer needs to understand and reflect on these. These include past experiences, irrational beliefs revisited, learned resilience, and faith in the context of hope, with forgiveness versus forgetting. The power of the unconscious again is reviewed, and problem ownership placed importantly besides feelings that can dominate, or inappropriate empathy that simply enables depression to continue.

Have you ever found yourself saying "I'm really depressed!"? Or maybe your good friend is known frequently to say something along those lines. Let's reflect here on what we might describe as the core issue we hear in these words.

More likely than not, the focus will involve strong negative feelings – those desperate feelings that so often can suddenly erupt, unbidden and at very inconvenient times. We can explore such feelings, be they within ourselves or our friend, to tease out likely synonyms that might explain more about those feelings. So now let's consider what better words may describe what is meant by "depressed".

Useful words other than saying: "I am depressed"

Jot down a list, which we'll come back to shortly.

Depression today is well known, accepted as a most debilitating "illness", affecting a huge proportion of our western society. Fortunately for many, however, being depressed has only a temporary impact. For example, consider the teenager's expression of "feeling depressed" while zits on the face dominate. It is really debilitating at the time, even if only obvious for a few months; but for many it can soon be accommodated, especially if effectively covered up! Or take

DOI: 10.4324/9781003474746-7

the young adult being depressed about a lack of friends, or a failed exam or a difficult job interview: unhappy circumstances that are relatively short-lived may indeed at the time *feel like* they will always be there, causing the person to react as if the problem will be permanent, can never change.

Having listened to such strong feelings with care and obvious genuine concern, we as carers are able to encourage reflection on the truthfulness or otherwise of their perception, and even to distract them enough to think about viable alternatives. A depressive episode thus becomes less dramatic, and eventually "lifts" with little intervention from anyone, especially when the feeling is understood by an important other. In fact, these very negative feelings can cause or be the catalyst as a positive motivator for change!

Is this phenomenon really to be accepted as depression? Or is this experience better considered as just the understandable reaction to the normal ups and downs in living, a reaction of an altered mood in response to the winds and storms of life? Is it realistic to expect a life free of any adversity or unhappiness? Is there a danger in considering any sense of unhappiness as a form of depression that implies a form of an illness, albeit mild?

Depression or something else?

Let's come back to your alternate list of "depressed" words: what does this list look like? I hope it demonstrates to you some of the more commonly used words that might better describe one's reaction to situations or circumstances that people naturally and realistically would prefer didn't exist – *being unhappy or glum; feeling miserable or sad; disheartened or discouraged; blue moods or just being lethargic, feeling down, despondent.*

I'm sure you identify with many of these descriptors, particularly when they are expressed about planned expectations that are seriously disappointed. Examples abound, like the weather that prevents a beautiful event, turning even alternatives into impossibilities; people who break commitments, leaving you feeling neglected, alone, or disillusioned about who you can trust; accidents or illness that change one's immediate plans, or more seriously impact future opportunities. The more serious any of these impacts are, the more inevitably some people will react with depressive symptoms that demand attention.
The global COVID19 pandemic experienced from 2020 onwards provides a well-identified basis for depression that has ongoing concerns, impacting even those not directly touched by it.

Of course, we may look up Wikipedia for a formal description, or consult the latest edition of the Diagnostic and Statistical Manual of Mental Illness (DSM) to get diagnostics from within a medical framework. Important though they are, such diagnostics can create a labelling trap. There is a need to understand how to use these descriptions that will enable someone who wants to move on through an episode and live a life free of that debilitating experience. It has been said that diagnostics are easy but devising effective treatment is another matter.

Here you may be reminded of someone you know who, when *diagnosed* with clinical depression, then lives as if that diagnosis is an inescapable life sentence. Remember Seligman's three Ps mentioned in Chapter 6: believing a problem is permanent, all pervasive, and to be taken personally. Such convictions can be a form of learned helplessness. Putting that into this context, you can see how quickly such beliefs may seem impossibly binding! Someone thus constrained may be surrounded by a small group of people who'd like to help, but most often they too feel there's nothing that can be done to bring relief. In fact, the sense of hopelessness can be quite infectious.

I recall one client who, after several years of tolerating her partner's more recent depression, admitted she feared becoming depressed herself. She decided to get some help, to prevent her from going down the same path.

Avril had known firsthand what depression looked like: her father had suffered from shellshock (the term given to those soldiers who returned from World War 1 damaged by their exposure to warfare). He'd had a limited capacity to live a "normal" life. His patience with people, things going wrong, and his angry frustration with his own inability to get a decent job that would provide for his family had left her super-sensitive to the moods now of her partner, Harry. You will recognise soldiers of later war experiences with many of those symptoms, usually labelled as suffering from PTSD – Post Traumatic Stress Disorder.[1]

As an unselfish, caring person, Avril for years had so carefully tried to meet Harry's needs, even before he expressed them. Now, however, she mainly sought to avoid the unpleasantness that would attend any neglect he perceived on her part. Harry had enjoyed being a leader and had expected this would always continue – until he was eventually displaced as a soccer team coach after serving 20 years, with no future prospect of taking on another team. He had found getting any job he liked impossible. The impact was felt financially, psychologically, and relationally – so everyone had to suffer!

Try to identify some precursors of Avril's present predicament: you may find at least three standouts. I will continue here with more about potential support options but hope you now take some moments to identify any potential blocks that may have contributed to Avril's own present inability to achieve a less stressed lifestyle, regardless of how Harry lived.

Write out a potential list of how *Avril's* past life may have explained how she felt so fearful about her own future, especially taking Harry and his depression into account.

Remember again: past experiences and beliefs can lead to present fears and anxieties.

It is not surprising to find that unremitting stress is the potential foundation on which future depression is built. One issue that dominated Avril's life was her conviction that she should be perfect: she must never make mistakes, and never *ever* say or do anything that might upset someone else!

Initially she was seriously challenged by rethinking the very possibility of not being perfect. Consider how this expectation naturally might extend to what she is likely to expect of others. But as her story unfolded it also became apparent that Avril had never learned to be assertive, and here you may need to think again of the discussion back in Chapter 2. Avril recognised that a serious adjustment was needed to her belief that good relationships depended on her correct or "perfect" behaviour, through which she had remained intensely committed to being compliant, a "Yes dear" person. Only then was she finally able to see that, in fact, much of her behaviour had actually *enabled* Harry's aggressive demands.

If you think about the small child whose parent does the same thing, permissively giving in, you will understand in that scenario the likely outcome: the child becomes obnoxiously selfish, the parent feels a victim, with life seeming to become increasingly out of control. With Avril ignoring her own needs when so focused on empathy with and for Harry's feelings, this circumstance had further confirmed *his own* feelings of the permanency of his current situation, with no positive possibilities for his future also seemingly endorsed by Avril's behaviour towards him.

Consider precursors to potential depression

Irrational beliefs[2] are often tenaciously maintained: but why, do you ask? You will remember that so often, feelings are hugely responsible for a person's conclusions about themselves or their situation that so often are not to be trusted. In Avril's case, her feelings of frustration about not being able to keep Harry happy were themselves being conflicted by her *previously* well-honed commitment to believing her own personal feelings didn't matter. Do you recognise the contradictions? Avril was confronted by internal conflict: how could she live with neglecting Harry's needs, while at the same time be cognisant at some level that she could not continue living with such unremitting stress? After all, she was now 60, and had hoped to enjoy an early retirement. Her reference to high blood pressure suggested that a medical reason had become the justification for her taking the advice given to seek help.

Resolving the internal conflict almost seemed more difficult than attempting to change the externally generated conflict with the man she had thought she should keep happy. Education about what we mean when we (wrongly) believe that we can make someone else happy was a useful focus. She knew as a parent what she had at least learned with her own children: that they each carried some responsibility in finding ways to enjoy life. When rethinking this truth, Avril reflected on how each of her three adult children was now variously succeeding within the context of their own generation.

Note how irrational beliefs contribute to feeling depressed.

As already mentioned in the context of changing behaviours, challenging irrational beliefs needs to go hand in hand with defining new beliefs that are compatible with those that bring internal peace. A technique sometimes called "chaining", found to be extremely useful and helpful for many clients caught by confusion, involves the asking of a series of questions about the behaviour that dominates a malformed belief system: "what does doing X or Y do for you?" In other words, we ask the person to drill down, to ask again after each response: "and what does THAT do for you . . . and then, what does THAT do for you?"

Try it, by answering a question about what motivates you to want to start a regular exercise programme? Maybe to feel good, or look good, or become more fit? . . . and to each answer you then ask: what does feeling/looking/being . . . do for you? Ultimately, we all want to be happier, don't we? Perhaps more satisfied, or more content at least?

Avril had faithfully served Harry well for a long time, believing that if she could make him happy, she would be too. Unfortunately, that belief was found to be flawed, for neither she nor her husband was happy. Some such beliefs had to be replaced, to provide a greater potential of achieving internal satisfaction and peace. Or at least, she needed to remove the internal war within: her need to oblige others being at the expense of another important part of her that knew life should be more than this!

Reflecting on the childhood experiences that had formed her long-held beliefs, now found wanting, was a good start. Having her also consider alternatives meant that Avril began to think of *herself* as taking responsibility for what her own future might look like. Because these alternative beliefs needed to be her own, owning them became an important motivator for making change possible. To replace the perfection belief, Avril learned to acknowledge and then adopt more realistic ones, such as: I am ok even when I make mistakes; when I allow *myself* to be imperfect, I become less critical of others; when I make mistakes, I am acknowledging I am human, fallible, so am less hard on myself, more relaxed.

I am sure you may quickly form some even more powerful alternative beliefs, some that are both tenable and helpful, avoiding stress-creating demands that are clearly self-destructive, both of relationships in general as well as of you personally.

Faith that counters irrational beliefs

Some of these beliefs may well also be formed for those with a commitment to a belief in there being a loving God who accepts individuals as they are, warts and all. Such faith has been shown to provide an empowering basis on which to dismiss feeling depressed, particularly about our personal inadequacies. Seligman himself supported the understanding of how important faith can be in overcoming negative views of self, shared in his book, *Learned Optimism*, though he admitted he did not personally hold such faith. For Avril, her early childhood faith became an adjunct to her finding greater support for a more positive perspective of herself, one that did not create internal irreconcilable conflicting beliefs.

When our irrational thoughts are replaced with reasonable, honest, and believable thought patterns, it is wonderful to see the palpable relief. So often, thoughts and their respective underlying negative beliefs result in a depressed mood which, when maintained for too long, can seem immutable, leading many to a dependence on drugs or simply on comfort food, to make them feel less despondent.

Distinguishing exogenous from endogenous depression

But you may be thinking: what about when our moods or feelings of despair are not simply based on specific identifiable irrational beliefs? It is useful here to consider those who clearly suffer from a mood disorder which is considered endogenous – that is, results from a physiological problem that relates to brain disorders over which the person has little agency. The endogenous and exogenous influences are often difficult to untangle. Mind–body understandings suggest that each can result from the other. No matter whether endogenous or exogenous, however, someone suffering from a depressive illness can be served well when their largely unconscious and negative thoughts, attitudes, and beliefs are reconfigured, reframed, bringing about a positive impact on the illness per se.

I am reminded of a client who had suffered a serious car accident which led to an ABI (Acquired Brain Injury). As a result, Philippa had experienced several psychotic episodes that ultimately required medical intervention. But she hated being on medication, resenting how her body felt because of weight gain associated with the medication, which contributed to her feeling lethargic (all this on top of eating inappropriately for comfort). This meant she also found it so difficult to complete the physical exercise she really needed.

Part of her learning to live again without feeling so overwhelmed by depression required her to understand that her brain was indeed an organ, a positive reframing of her negative perspective on the one small but important part of her that was now malfunctioning. Philippa completely understood this when asked how she felt about people who suffered with a kidney disease or from heart problems that required lifelong dependence on medication. She then became less affected by depressive thoughts about being on anti-psychotic drugs. She also became accepting of the need to retrain her focus towards positive beliefs, deliberately practising ones that formed good attitudes towards worthwhile behaviours that could minimise the effects of the necessary drugs. This included Philippa making a disciplined commitment to physical exercise and dietary requirements, thus avoiding further psychotic episodes and the likelihood of future diabetes due to being overweight.

We will return shortly to thinking of other examples of people whose depression was exogenous, and furthermore, not simply *irrationally* based. After all, it is understandable that a realist, as one who sees the world as it really is, may often feel pessimistic about future human efforts to live in an idealistic, perfect world, when all around them the world is falling apart! But this notion introduces other elements that demonstrate how we may assist those experiencing depression, by learning to better *manage* their depression. The powerful effect of dismissing unhelpful beliefs should never be minimised.

In the case of Avril above, her own revised sense of helplessness in relation to Harry was soon part of the relief that was offered to *him*, with Avril becoming the partner who no longer *enabled* his total dependence on her for his own future. Yes, he continued to benefit from antidepressant medication for some time, but his general mood gradually improved, joining Avril in some of her own new behaviours that brought her much joy, and some important distractions for Harry. She finally had accepted it was appropriate to want to enjoy life, even to take up new hobbies which did not include Harry. But yes, Avril's depressive and fearful thoughts had been quite understandable, so in my role I needed in part to help normalise such feelings, given where their life together was heading, unless and until important changes were made. Any such depression is referred to as exogenous depression, as being related to and reactively caused by unmanaged outside stressors.

Identify external situations/circumstances
that create negative feelings.

You can see how important it is then to face any reactive responses to disturbing external factors, and to particularly challenge those beliefs that have proved to be unhelpful in dealing with trauma. Avril was faced with certain generational patterns of living, first modelled to her by her own mother, and which she in turn had been modelling to her only daughter. She also was able to reflect on the unacceptable behaviours of others that had influenced her thinking. She reported that her two sons had rejected their father, thus were more independent of family expectations, though some issues were still problematic for her daughter.

Here you may reflect on families you know where depression is even considered to be inherited: as if, being genetic, the *behavioural* expressions of that depressed way of thinking cannot be helped. There may well be physiological and personality *similarities* that make the inheritance possibility more plausible, but the old question of how much is influenced by nature or nurture[3] remains a necessary unknown. Individual differences again highlight this ongoing research conundrum.

Depression – inherited, modelled, even cultural?

Others will sometimes suggest that depression, as an illness, be conceptualised as a disease. With this comes an implied notion of its potentially even being contagious! While we may dismiss this when it is called out, this belief could be defensible when we see group work with depressed people which, as mentioned earlier in Chapter 6, unless managed well, tends to embellish the symptoms rather than reduce them. Interpersonal contagion we can also readily observe in social media today, especially obvious in relation to conspiracy theorists.

Evidence abounds of how the acceptance of cultural beliefs and attitudes concerns even the impact of trauma on people, with claims that, as a result, depression alone often explains and even excuses all manner of unacceptable behaviours. This understanding of depression can also extend to a person's lack of interest in helping at home, say with basic chores, in finding or staying in a job, or sadly, it can even extend to allowances made in court for criminal offences.

I am reminded of a colleague who reacted strongly to hearing about the lived experiences of three young adult medicos we knew well. After completing temporary work placements in an isolated African community, these doctors reported how well the indigenous peoples had accepted the death of one child and even subsequent children, considering such traumas are simply what life brings. The same surprised colleague then said: "They should be taught about the stages of the grieving process, so they can take themselves through those stages and cope better, avoiding the likelihood for experiencing PTSD!"

Was this an imposition of western culture-based psychology, perhaps? What do you think?

Learned resilience

At the heart of their culture, these African people lived with realistic expectations about life in their world that enabled them to openly express and accept their grief before moving on. Such a culture also demonstrates that humans do have a great many different and effective ways of building a capacity for endurance and resilience.

Depression often results from beliefs that focus on considering a glass half empty, as if permanent, pervasive, and personal. Resilience needs hope. Hope comes from focusing on the half-full rather than the half-empty glass. This is most observable when, after acknowledging problems and pain as real but transitory – not all-pervasive and not personal – people are encouraged to find things that motivate them to achieve new hopes and dreams, in spite of grief and loss.

Reconsider Albert Ellis's Ten Irrational Beliefs

I cannot emphasise strongly enough, however, that in listening to the stories of people we seek to help, we need to be clear about the positive potentials associated with taking personal responsibility for one's own thoughts and behaviours. I also would like to reiterate the importance of encouraging others to evaluate Ellis's Rational Emotive Behaviour Therapy (REBT), for the veracity and the rationality of any destructive beliefs that can be so debilitating. Perhaps you would benefit from looking up on the web the list of well-defined destructive Irrational Beliefs posited by REBT.[4] Such lists at least in part can inform some of your own beliefs that may warrant appropriate new alternatives.

Here again we reflect on how feelings, unless accepted and affirmed as a person's truth, can make it nigh impossible to move beyond and through ill-formed and long-standing irrational or unhelpful attitudes and beliefs. This is the case irrespective of whether the person is suffering from exogenous or endogenous depression. The potentially depressive dark cloud over an individual's ability to think clearly needs to be lifted. Supportive concern takes a real commitment by the helper to stay long enough with the suffering person to earn the opportunity and the right to encourage a move forward.

Be honest about your own personal capacity to do this; only then will you be more able to avoid unnecessary stress, particularly when success is elusive, potentially suggesting that *you* are a failure! Referring the client on then becomes a positive option, for both client and carer.

This throws us back to thinking again about *problem ownership*, mentioned in Chapter 4. Regardless of who may have modelled the behaviour, or how long it has been a comfortable part of an individual's pattern of living, owning the problem for oneself is so crucial to enable moving on.

Another client may help to clarify what I am trying to convey here. This man, Colin, was a returned soldier, who finally at 55 had accepted that he could no longer maintain a job because of his debilitating depressive moods. Fortunately, society in general acknowledges the awfulness of war but sadly without making a commitment to cease making war the only resolution to conflict! We have also seen how war impacts not only the individuals involved but also their families, and often for generations.

However, in Colin's case, when as a young 20-year-old he had been conscripted for the war in Vietnam, his life's plan of becoming a builder was seriously interrupted. Not just by the two-and-a-half years taken from him, but by the recovery period after he returned. This partly resulted from physical damage when his wounds took so long to heal. But the unseen and thus unrecognised psychological impact had never been acknowledged. Such scarring lingers internally and yet is often far more devastating than a physical injury, in terms of the well-being of all in the family.

Take a moment: consider how typically people with ***hidden*** *physical disabilities, like deafness for example, report being treated less well than those who are more obviously disabled.*

Interesting, isn't it: those with vision loss or other physical limitations (thus needing a seeing eye dog or wheelchair or artificial limbs) are more likely to receive patience and attention, as they are more obvious. For the internal struggles arising from *invisible* debilitating traumas, there is often little sympathy or understanding, not only from others but also as regards the sufferer's personal acceptance. In our culture, hiding pain is often lauded as demonstrating positive characteristics, of stoicism or even some sort of heroism. Many a sufferer has reported guilt at expressing how they are feeling. Reflect here on what role you may find appropriate as a potential support person.

Visible physical injuries compared to inner, psychological traumas

Returning to Colin, he had reportedly tried to complete an apprenticeship when his physical injuries were deemed medically healed. But it hadn't taken long into that training course before his reactive depression became more obvious.

Initially his young partner Bertha found him becoming often insensitive and short-tempered, self-preoccupied, and difficult to live with. Then before too long, she reported this as having extended into his exploding unpredictably at their children, with little apparent cause or knowledge of the triggers for the episode.

Bertha began protecting the children by defending Colin with comments like "Daddy is tired – just be a bit quieter" and this had ended with the children becoming quite fearful of upsetting him. They couldn't understand why he was always such a "bear with a sore head", but they soon learned not to bring their friends home.

Finally, to escape the tensions, the teenaged children left home. While it relieved *their* tensions, their mother was then left alone, trying to keep the peace while living with a disturbed isolated man. The children no longer were there to blame or provide an avenue for his venting, so his focus turned to reacting to the demands of his workplace. With increased belligerence towards his undeserving workmates, Colin's boss suggested early retirement – but how would he cope?

As things deteriorated, his wife finally admitted ultimate despair: she'd had enough, so in the end *he* was left to suffer alone. Gradually alcohol had become his means of deadening the internal pain, a preferred way of self-medicating that meant even his dreams were not remembered. Eventually diagnosed with the common mental illness of war, suffering from PTSD, Colin was given appropriate anti-depressants and a disability pension from the Australian Government Department of Veterans' Affairs (DVA). He was finally enabled to start working part-time, but then only for himself – being his own boss meant he could actually keep going, pacing himself and with no one to argue with. He could now choose when and where he worked, and if people annoyed him, he simply downed tools and went elsewhere.

Reactive depression – powerful and potentially destructive

For another five years, Colin survived reasonably well and built up a tidy bank balance . . . until a decision to join a relative in a small business venture brought him undone. After discovering he had financially been taken advantage of, Colin became fired up with accumulated anger. This emerged with a determination to end it all. Colin had taken his gun, sat outside his relative's home most of the night, trying to find the courage to shoot his relative and then himself. Through the haze of intoxication, he remembered enough about the values instilled by his parents in his upbringing to know this was a terrible, reactive plan, one that could not leave him with anything but feeling enormous guilt should he not succeed in killing himself. The angst of not being able to pull the trigger on himself, even if he'd shot the relative, finally took over. He went home in anguish, promising himself he would now seek the help he'd been offered years before. The event was the trigger point (pun intended) for him to own up to facing a deeply destructive personal crisis.

Over the next few sessions, I listened to the immediate near-disaster, and after Colin had shared his war experiences, he began to not only understand but accept how he'd succumbed to the effects of silently carrying the traumas of war. Part of supporting him involved helping him realise that he was in company with many other fine men and women who had travelled equally lonely journeys. Blaming others for how he felt had been his only resource, while maintaining his denial of unresolved emotions. As this realisation progressed, some of his angst was magnified by becoming aware that he himself had generated a large part of his present circumstances, a matter that needed to be worked through realistically, without trivialising or excusing, yet also without being judgemental. Only then could he contemplate better ways of dealing with his underlying, mostly ignored feelings.

You ask how his story ended: were his marriage and finances restored? Well, this was never part of his goal, nor should it ever be that of the counsellor. However, what *was* restored was a sense of self that had long been lost, along with a belief in himself that he could manage, and without betraying his real desire to be someone of integrity. He came to accept that living alone was quite comforting, allowing him choices about whether he needed company or not.

So how was this achieved? Put briefly, much of it can be attributed to his coming to the end of himself. Going back to thinking about what he had lost, learning to forgive others as he learnt to love and accept himself. Part of Colin's healing came through learning to take responsibility for caring for his own physical needs. A plan to exercise regularly was committed to, while he also decided to turn his erstwhile drinking habit into something he could enjoy. Yes, he could enjoy the very thing that had become part of his downfall, but only when he accepted being responsible for limiting his intake! Colin firstly learnt how to make his own beer, and such a process was not only enjoyed but valued – so he drank far less! And there was an unexpected beneficial consequence from the beer-making itself: it became a social enterprise. There is nothing like good friendships that form around enjoying working on a project together. Instead of drinking being merely a means to the end of drowning his feelings, beer became a subject that precipitated much-needed social sharing in the tasting and mutual enjoyment of it. So it was that he learned to be careful, to be patient, and to start trusting a small number of friends who were willing for him to call them up, should he risk breaking his commitment to those tasks that provided a potent balm to his injured self.

Forgiveness – forgetting? Or a new perspective?

I'd like to give you a brief insight into another Vietnam War veteran seen over a period of months. Garry needed someone to know his story, to understand why he'd had to go bush, to get away from the noise and bustle that simply amplified his internal distress. He refused to accept his psychiatrist's diagnosis of being depressed, though he had agreed to early retirement on a returned serviceman's pension. He gradually reported some enjoyment getting up in the morning, growing his own vegetables, and taking his dog for long walks on his acreage.

After sharing many elements of his overseas service that still invaded his habitually broken sleep, keeping him very tired, Garry committed to writing his story. This activity became a valuable part of his day. Several weeks later, he brought me a copy – many pages of written memories about his time in the army, much of which he reported had now brought him to healing tears. A final couple of sessions were used to reinforce regular relaxation, particularly when he was disturbed by memories.

Six months went by before suddenly he attended for a one-off session. I asked what brought him in that day, and his answer surprised me. "I just need to be forgiven", he said, as his huge frame settled deeper into the chair. He looked forlorn, unlike previously when he had mostly appeared to be in control while speaking without a lot of feeling. I checked if there was anything he had done recently that he regretted, but no, it was a personal new insight. Having been a young, innocent, naïve young man at the call-up time was no longer perceived as an adequate excuse. He now felt conflicted, even tormented, convinced he should have been a conscientious objector!

During his initial sessions, Garry had shared a little of what life was like *before* his compulsory time in the army, which had led to his hopes of becoming a teacher being permanently dashed. On release from army life he had simply completed a trade school opportunity, before finally becoming a greens' keeper for golf courses, over many years. He now briefly recalled parts of his army time again for me, highlighting with obvious regret the reason why he now needed to feel forgiven – things he had seen, actions of others that he had simply turned a blind eye to. He recalled how he had often felt angry at his own lack of compunction to speak up.

I sensed that I needed to find a point of his beliefs to leverage against the guilt. After a slow start, I gently asked whether he believed in a God who loves and forgives. "Oh, definitely yes", he said, "otherwise I wouldn't still be here today." He had been brought up in a Christian family, and that experience had taught him good ways of living, but he acknowledged he had not thought much about God until recently. He wished he had accepted imprisonment back in 1970,[5] rather than allowing himself to be part of what he now believed had been absolutely criminal. His remorse was evident, the sadness and obvious regret accompanying his request, stating he needed to be forgiven.

It seemed strange that he had come to me for this gift, though obviously he felt safe enough to know he would not feel judged. It was therefore a privilege for me to offer my understanding, with an assurance of forgiveness that I believe reflected my own belief: there is nought we can do that the patient creative God would not forgive, given Jesus' claim to have made forgiveness available for all through his ultimate sacrifice.

He sat with eyes closed as if in relaxation while I shared biblically based words of comfort. After sitting quietly for several minutes, I recall his sitting up straight, followed by his smiled thanks, before quietly saying, "I really needed to hear that!" I again checked briefly with him about life in general, and got the clear indication that no other issues were worrying him. He reported feeling quite content, that he was satisfied he needed no further counselling – "unless something comes up", he said as he smiled then quietly left. Empowered, it now seemed, to live the simple life, without suffering from the self-condemnation he had experienced for many years, but only recently had faced. As found by all who practise forgiveness, it does not mean forgetting, but it does allow the hurts, the mistakes, and any guilt felt to be put into a different perspective, one that more effectively enables one to learn from the past but not be destroyed by it.

We may not always understand what a person needs, or why their perception of what they need is so important to them. But we can be quite surprised by the changes made as a result of a person sharing their innermost concerns. We can't make predictions about the next stage of life that may yet impact or become important to that same person. Some may seek your ear for a completely different reason another time in the future, with the earlier work having created important stepping stones. But our own personal integrity is essential if our support is to be trusted to provide a meaningful and positive contribution to a person's journey.

The power of self-instructions

Have you ever reflected on some of the things of the past that have seemed almost inconsequential at the time, but that, in hindsight, you recognise to have made an important impact to the life you now live? For some people, new reflections on those things can reveal what has now caught up with them, creating a fresh understanding about the events that led to depression. Think about your own life: the influences on who you are, how you feel about yourself, about life in general. This next example may stimulate a curiosity for reflection on how "this connects with that", particularly about those connections that only the individual involved is able to make sense of.

An interesting referral came from a local doctor, who recommended some therapy for a lady who he said was quite depressed. Some months earlier Gaye had experienced being in a coma, after a routine operation to remove a grumbling appendix that had irregularly caused pain. The surgeon reported no physical reasons for the coma which had lasted well over a week, during which finally her family had been called in potentially to say their goodbyes. The perplexed doctors could find no explanation of what had happened and were not expecting her to recover.

As Gaye eventually reported to me, she had suddenly and unexpectedly regained consciousness, with no serious physiological side effects apparent, but still could not return to work, feeling distressed, depressed, and otherwise very unwilling to return to normal life. She lamented lacking her previous vitality. After my probing questions, she reported being quite fearful: an undiagnosed illness might suddenly plunge her again into a coma. Her GP had referred her for some relaxation sessions, hoping for some psychological insights that might help her depression.

Listening to her story suggested to me that there must be some underlying rationale to explain the marked pre- and post-operative differences Gaye described about herself. She had never been a "depressed" person: she was rather outgoing, usually enthusiastic and energetic. It seemed that she had simply shut down, so Gaye needed to experience a deep session of both muscle and mind relaxation, before a more verbal understanding of her present sense of depression could be considered.

Parts work – engaging the subconscious

In common everyday talk, people can often readily identify inner conflicts as if from different parts of their mind. How often do we hear someone say something like: "A part of me wants to do A, but another part B . . ." This can be leveraged in what has been called "parts work", drawn from Gestalt Therapy[6] where the technique seeks to bring to consciousness the activity of different parts of our unconscious mind. With her being in a relaxed mode, I asked Gaye to recall how she had been before her operation and illness. No problem was raised from any part of her mind – and all parts reported being quite glad about the result achieved by the appendix removal. I then asked her to identify and invite an incredible but unconsciously controlling part of her to remember if anything had happened immediately before going into hospital that caused the shutdown. It responded with a startled "wake up" reaction, causing her to suddenly open her eyes to say: "Oh, my gosh, I remember now! I remember saying to my work mates on the Tuesday prior to the op, that come Friday, I will do a complete shut down, so I won't have to do absolutely *anything* for more than a whole week!"

The power of self-talk mentioned in Chapter 1 was again highlighted to me – we don't always appreciate how we may have been affected by this internal capability to influence or change us, even though it may be completely forgotten. Further relaxation for Gaye meant we could quietly reflect on what had happened, when that subconscious part of her had quite *literally* taken on board her happily expressed instruction. A child-like part of her mind (one that is often observed to be uninhibited by deep thinking) now expressed real remorse, almost like a child caught out doing something it shouldn't have. It quickly reassured Gaye it would never do something like that again! At that point, it was important to facilitate an interchange with other parts of her mind, too, so that in future they would check for agreement that any course of action would be negotiated, and quite consciously decided on by Gaye herself.

Unbelievable, I'm sure you think, and so I would have thought, prior to this, but along with later examples, it proves again just how amazing our minds are. How fearfully yet wonderfully made! Two more appointments were set to check how Gaye was coping, and the second one was cancelled, she then being back at work and reporting "feeling back to normal".

REFLECTIVE EXERCISES

Check out how some of your regular expressions are evidence of unconscious self-talk – of internal, automatic self-instructions that lead to either good or less positive outcomes. Write them down. Become consciously aware of how repetitive they may have become.

For example: I never like doing . . . I always say . . . I don't ever do X, because it never works! Affirm those which are worthwhile keeping, but do challenge yourself to reconsider whether you would benefit from rethinking certain internal statements you live by. Be prepared to abort those which are not helpful.

The next chapter will provide more real-life circumstances that may convince you again of the power of (even forgotten) self-talk!

Notes

1 PTSD is often appropriately differentiated today as ASD, Acute Stress Disorder, or, alternatively, as an Adjustment Disorder, suggestive of depression associated with significant personal life changes.
2 Irrational beliefs can form into dysfunctional schemas, explored in Chapter 16.
3 You may like to look up some good articles about the nature/nurture dilemma.
4 REBT: core beliefs as self-defeating thoughts and emotions. See various resources on the internet for "REBT Irrational Beliefs".
5 Look up conscription and the Vietnam War, 1962–75.
6 This technique is best understood as an application of Gestalt Therapy. There is much information readily online to give you a useful understanding of this and similar techniques.

Chapter 8

More on depression

Depression calls out many questions around its treatment, including when medication may be warranted, and perhaps even before certain forms of depression are effectively confronted. Other treatment/co-treatment options in relation to individual debilitating depressive symptoms sometimes include group therapy, with some cautions discussed about potential limitations. A systems theory approach uses the illustration of a mobile, where balancing explains the interpersonal forces within groups experiencing change. The impact of memories is explored, particularly in relation to unresolved grief. The trusted listener who is comfortable with emotional release becomes part of the process towards the lifting of depression, especially when this is married to a deeper understanding of personality issues that may have contributed to a serious lack of resilience. Reference to energy gainers versus energy drainers is also presented as additional insights into understanding depression.

We commonly refer to depression as possibly being present when a person consistently experiences low mood, finds it difficult to wake up in the mornings, lacks motivation to get out of bed, or conversely can't get to sleep, even when clearly very tired. As you may have reflected with regard to the few examples in the previous chapter, there are sometimes good reasons for a person to feel depressed.

Recalled memories can help explain depressive behaviours.

Understandably, unless that reason is understood, or circumstances re-evaluated, getting over the state of depression may seem impossible. Feelings that relate to a sense of self-worth, guilt feelings that remain hidden, unmet needs that are perceived to be all-important – many or all of these may indicate that an individual's mind is so clouded that antidepressant medication may seem to be warranted.

DOI: 10.4324/9781003474746-8

Caution: medication for depression

Before moving on to specific examples, I believe a cautionary note about the diagnosis of depression is necessary here. Even as I write, a well-researched article cites some alarming statistics about the dispensing of anti-depressants in Australia,[1] making it one of the highest-prescribing nations in the world. This article points to a lack of due deference to the clinical guidelines which relate to the severity of the reported depression *as a psychiatric diagnosis*, so that too often there is a quick resorting to prescribing anti-depressants when they are not needed. The author writes that "overprescribing antidepressants is a symptom of our lack of attention to the social determinants of mental health. . . . there may be a medical explanation but [it] is most often found in the person's struggles . . . [which requires] looking at other ways to improve their mental health." In other words, care is needed to uncover the external issues that have contributed to the person's depressive mood. He goes on to clarify both the troubling side effects of anti-depressants, the significant problems of withdrawal symptoms, and other issues related to their long-term use.

Some important research has clearly established the effectiveness of medication *when coupled with cognitive and behavioural therapies*, over and above medication used alone; the latter option often means the depressive behaviour becomes interminable. Practitioners have also found that *without* some supportive medication, however, a seriously depressed individual at times may have great difficulty taking personal responsibility for making the necessary cognitive psychological changes. Medication *can* pave the way to greater clarity of thinking. Used appropriately, medication can enable the disheartened sufferer, feeling so thought-disordered, to finally begin to unravel the real issues. This usually involves finding the cognitive and emotional factors that are making significant, if not the main, contributions to their depressed mental state. When the brain is less confused or muddled, a number of different therapeutic approaches can then be utilised to achieve relief from depressive thoughts. This process can allow repressed memories to become more available.

But in Gaye's case discussed in Chapter 7, the need for medication was not deemed necessary, so that together we were able to effectively challenge her negative thoughts and cognitions in the context of digging into her unconscious. As with many people experiencing depression, this included making both a necessary cognitive and behavioural shift to achieve wellness, including a commitment to regular exercise.

Much like taking painkillers for painful physical ailments that simply required attention, long-term dependency on medication alone for psychological pain is often problematic. Without the *mediating* power of thoughtful sharing about the basis of disturbing beliefs and their associated behaviours, medication may simply mask the negative feelings and can seriously negate a much-needed sense of self-efficacy.

Being able to make effective longer-term changes is related to a capacity for taking ownership of the problem. Whether or not to take medication should be considered in relation to achieving that goal. Have a look back to Chapter 4, where problem ownership is recognised as essential for empowerment. And, from Chapter 7, remember the veteran soldier Colin, or even Harry who had modelled on his own father and had developed a dependency on his wife. Both men had to learn to take personal responsibility for their behaviours, and then could create opportunities for developing their own resilience.

A personal sense of being in control is an essential cognitive element in overcoming depression, enabling an individual to confidently challenge and change erroneous or unhealthy values and beliefs.

Social and group dynamics

One-on-one sharing of debilitating thoughts is important. But sometimes it can be helpful to share with a group, especially with others suffering similar issues. Group work is often considered more cost-effective, and potentially provides a supportive context for moving on towards personal well-being. But some caution is needed if this approach is to be considered a serious option for overcoming depression. As mentioned earlier, if it is not well handled, I have seen shared despair simply plunge each participant deeper into their own despair.

Overcoming depression is never simple or easy, exacerbated by elements of the depression itself. This is particularly so when a depression has become associated with strongly held habitual maladaptive thinking schemas that control day-to-day living, and in which other people have also become enmeshed. More of Schema Therapy will be reflected on in Chapter 16. Such patterns of behaviour become so difficult to break – and for the associated "helping" people, too, who themselves can become entrapped, even comfortable with how it is. When that occurs, the current attitude of "that's life; it is what it is" is heard as a throwaway line, so often seriously and fatalistically delivered! Genuinely concerned people may also wind up unwittingly providing a pay-off for staying depressed, for example through the well-intentioned special extra care given to the one feeling depressed. This pay-off is referred to as secondary gain, mentioned as what became Sabina's fallback position in Chapter 6. But in this context of social supports, secondary gain can mean that the extra care/attention does not contribute to the depression itself, but can indeed serve to maintain it.

Social interactions often take on a life of their own, variously effective depending on how much people either accept or reject the sufferer's behaviours. But more formal group times have the potential to make individuals feel less isolated, more accepted because of the group dynamics that form through similarity of problems.

Mobile balance

In group work we can see some evidence that supports the picture of hanging mobiles, developed in what is known as Systems Theory. Here the mobile has been used to represent the interpersonal dynamics within a family, as part of family therapy, or group of friends or associates in a workplace, for example.

A complex mobile is beautiful when it is well-balanced, and every part moves smoothly. But if you change the weight or position of just one part of the mobile, you will observe an unevenness that can cause a serious imbalance, even to the point that it becomes a very different mobile, though the various parts still somehow hang together. Likewise, there is a natural movement of individuals within groups to maintain or regain balance, either by themselves moving to counterbalance someone else's changes, or by trying to hold back the individual seeking to change, simply to keep their own position in the group stable. When these groups are well-managed, a purposeful interchange between depressed people can be quite beneficial. On the other hand, the group itself can resent or feel threatened by any individual who starts to make the positive changes that others can't, won't, or are not ready to make.

A good example is seen in a classroom, when support given to the "naughty" child changes their behaviour to the extent that they become thought of as the "good" kid. Consequently, that child threatens the erstwhile "teacher's pet", so the balance of power changes!

Much of such sabotage is completely unwitting, and individuals can be horrified when their actions are brought to light. The facilitator of such a group needs to be aware of what is happening, and competent to channel or moderate the disruptive interactions occurring.

A cautionary note: resistance to change from within a group can be quite powerful in one way or another. Don't ever undertake leading such a group without having the necessary skills and personal integrity. You may like to look up the fascinating area of Systems Theory in psychology, included under other titles such as Family Systems theory/therapy.

Depression always demands deep understanding.

Feelings of depression should *never* be dismissed as silly, attention-seeking, or treated as passing follies, even though secondary gain or other social influences may be contributing.

I cannot leave this chapter without reference to Donna, a very sad lady, late 30s, whose expressed evidence of depression included insisting that she had killed her baby. Even her husband had not believed her story, with the result that her claims had never been treated as serious or rational but were rather seen as psychotic inventions. Such ideas were expressed to her psychiatrists, along with numerous other highly emotional but mostly negative mood statements about her life. Much of what Donna claimed was dismissed as delusional. Her emotionally unstable state of mind was deemed evidence that her claims were not to be treated seriously! Her husband of several years had little insight into his wife's emotional needs, so had increasingly just given in to her victim-mentality which demanded her whims simply be granted, spoilt by being given nice things to try to make her happy.

This deeply unhappy lady had experienced years of trialling various antidepressants, with no medications providing relief other than making her want to sleep most of her days, doped up and incapable of cognitive reasoning. Donna had not received any psychotherapeutic treatment options either, as these were thought to be inadequate for her entrenched psychiatric symptoms. Frequently hospitalised, in the early 1980s she was administered many rounds of shock treatment (a treatment of the day) in a country facility. Her quality of life was severely impacted. Donna's despairing husband had finally asked that she be seen by a psychologist when next released from hospital for a home visit, hoping for some temporary relief, through relaxation at least.

During that visit, with careful questioning that implied her story would be believed, Donna revealed that she had never been asked about *when* she had done this terrible act. Her response was incredibly enlightening. Though delivered very emotionally, Donna was clearly able to articulate her distress as she spoke about an enforced abortion at 16. Her parents had found it too embarrassing to allow her to keep the child. She had not received any counselling about her grief and loss, and the traumatic episode was simply pushed into a closed book. Her marriage some years later had brought no children, and only increased her depth of depression. Time had simply kept open a tragic book.

The end of her story, you ask? Initially Donna expressed great relief at revealing her regret, her feelings of guilt. In a long emotional session, her newly found genuine positive response lay in accepting that really the guilt was not hers to hold, nor was the responsibility for what had taken place. She said this was the first time in her adult life she had felt happy!

Sadly, the happiness she expressed was short-lived. Her new and completely unexpected positive state of mind was medically misunderstood, interpreted as being related to the shock treatment of the prior weeks. Back in care, another bout of that same treatment meant she had no memory of the affective and cognitive understanding gained through the brief REBT, with the emotional relief she had experienced totally obliterated. Tragically, we learnt some weeks later that she had given up hope and taken her own life. No one at the time had any knowledge of her planned escape, or how deeply depressed she had been.

Regardless of the possibility that certain memories are distorted, delusional, or not real, if we are to help resolve such wrongly based beliefs, the personal stories revealed need to be dealt with *as if* they are real, for to the sufferer, they *are* real. In the context of seeking to bring wholeness and wellbeing, psychological insights need to be differentiated from the focus of legal and compensational inquiries.

Take responsibility – but only for what is under our control.

I have shared a weighty example here that you may find quite disturbing, but it demonstrates an important and truthful reality. We can never *guarantee* great outcomes, and *our* part in restoring health and well-being is but a part. Much of what we do in supporting people requires teamwork and collaboration – and even that sometimes can fail. This is indeed a humbling reality, but one that can also ultimately provide great relief: we should *never* take responsibility for what is not really under our control.

In fairness, I need to comment here that this case study reports a problem of the older use of shock treatment that at the time was relatively primitive, being reliant on general memory loss that accompanied the treatment. This may explain why Donna had no memory of the therapy that had brought a temporary relief. Who can say whether today, with improved neurological accuracy of treatment options, and also with a greater emphasis on interdisciplinary health provider collaboration, the inclusion of a psychological treatment plan now available may have had a very different outcome.

Unresolved grief that develops into depression

To continue this chapter on a more positive note, another example of someone experiencing depression may give us a more optimistic perspective on this ubiquitous health issue. After the birth of her second child, Marion was advised to get help, having been diagnosed at her community health centre as suffering from postnatal depression (PND), also reported as Postpartum Depression (PPD), which in Australia is reportedly thought to impact as many as up to 20 percent of women giving birth. Marion was really struggling to care for her baby, let alone her active two-year-old. She was given full-time care in a psychiatric ward for several days, then sent home on medication, but after many weeks she expressed concern that she was not coping any better. A friend suggested that some psychological help was worth trying.

> *What sort of questions are you now aware of that may demand answers? Make a list before reading on.*

Good questions provide important information

Remember, background questions are always important: those which identify how life was *before* the presenting problem. Some questions may lead to identifying when such low feelings began, and to understand the circumstances surrounding such feelings.

In Marion's case, she reported a loving husband, and a happy time experienced during the first two years of her son's life. Immediately after her daughter's arrival, however, Marion said things had gone pear-shaped. We needed to explore those details, to discover what that picture really looked like. She described how routines had suddenly gone out the door; there were toys and mess everywhere; she had no ability to organise her day so that preparing the main meal was always left to her husband after he returned from work. Marion needed to reflect on how she had managed with the advent of her first child. She now recognised that he had been a breeze baby – slept well, fed well, and had given her plenty of time to be her natural organised self. But her baby girl was very different: almost the opposite to her little boy in every regard. And now, what little time for herself she'd experienced *before* the second child had now became non-existent, made especially stressful with a very active toddler also demanding any spare time she had!

Individual needs that past history can reveal

Further reflection with Marion revealed a thoughtful lady who had always needed a lot of space to think, time to read, either to escape or make sense of the stressors that could at times overwhelm her. In addition, questions that related to further back in her pre-marriage life gave us both new insights about why she now felt so low: revealing, in "Les Mis" terms, "a grief that can't be spoken". Marion recalled a time when as a young teenager, she had had to say goodbye to her much-loved Mum, and recalled subsequent months of "trying to be brave". That resulted in her determining she would never allow herself to express her grief to others, for fear of not being able to keep going. She had learnt to keep up a bubbly happy face, and this resolution had largely served her well. It worked while life was kept simple, with only few things taken on that would otherwise have stretched her capacity to be super-organised. Her husband was earning a good income, so she no longer needed to keep up her stressful, complex job previously enjoyed. Clearly Marion had, until the second child arrived, enjoyed a fairly luxurious lifestyle, with her need for order and quietness easily maintained.

> *On top of the current issues that were created by the addition of another child, can you hear the various crucial elements that had long been ignored? Spend a few minutes jotting these down, before you go on reading.*

If you've re-read some of the cases mentioned earlier in relation to depression, you may realise it is rare for depression to present as an issue in isolation. In other words, the previously mentioned cumulative effect is common, and your own life experiences may confirm this to be true. So, when Marion shared her story of losing her mother, *and* her consequent determination to not give in to grief, it was possible to begin to see a way forward for this naturally very capable but feeling person. Giving her a safe place to sob was so appreciated and welcomed by Marion, accompanied by an assurance that crying is a God-given release of emotions, even crucial if we are to experience restorative healing.

Personality differences require understanding

Subsequent sessions enabled me to further engage her more realistically in assessing her own personality. As revealed by one inventory (the Myers-Briggs Type Indicator [MBTI][2]), she realised that her personality type, very different from her sister's, helped explain much of her "depression". As a warmly creative, emotional being, she had largely thought that if she just pretended, all would be well. She reflected on her older sibling who was happy to live in a mess with her children and had frequently told her she should just let things be, not worry so much! Understanding was required about her individual needs, and for these to be accepted and embraced, rather than resented or thought of as indicating some personal limitation, or a failure to be responsible.

Energy drainers and energy gainers

I'm sure you will be pleased to know that Marion recovered from her postnatal depression, and more quickly than even her husband had expected. Her unexplored grief, together with the relevance of not having a mum she could call on, was now thoughtfully reconsidered as part of who she was, as well as how she now felt. Caring for her two children had really made it necessary for her to confront some unmet needs she had previously not understood. It was important to give herself permission to treat her specific needs for tidiness and cleanliness, along with quiet times to experience much needed energy *gainers*, in the face of the energy *drainers* surrounding her.

Such personal understanding gave her permission to allow her very inner being to be respected and cared for. Practical activities, for example, were not naturally easy for her, so relief from some of these allowed her to "catch her wind", to enjoy a quiet reflective time and some creative thinking. This enabled a refreshing time for her to escape the here and now into another world, restoring the energy to keep doing the things life now demanded of her. This new possibility was allowed for by a house cleaner while things settled, and regular times for child minding, even if only for a few hours each week. Some small lifestyle changes were incredibly reassuring. Simply by expressing her deeply masked depressed feelings about herself, Marion could in fact bring about insights and opportunity to appropriately resolve the energy drainers, now exposed as unmet needs, with much-needed regained energy. In addition, both she and her husband now better understood her personality, with her associated personal needs, quite different from his, and now better accommodated.

REFLECTIVE EXERCISES

1. It is vital to review our own behaviours, checking on any that may be childish or unhelpful, or perhaps not really understood: but is this something you find challenging? I don't ask why, but it may be good to answer the question: what do you gain by ignoring the issue? When this is honestly considered and acted on, you will know *experientially* more about what may be helpful for others to understand about themselves.
2. You might also spend some time reflecting on what sort of things *you* are likely to feel depressed about. What do you do with them? Dwell on them and feel really depressed? Ignore them and pretend they don't matter?
3. What alternative thoughts do you have to prevent situations or circumstances from overwhelming everyday life? What enables you to effectively explore resilience for when tough times hit?
4. What activities are energy *drainers* for you? And what energy *gainers* do you actively engage in, to keep that necessary balance, to deal with the problems associated with "all work and no play"?

5. Do you hold any unhelpful or destructive personal beliefs that perhaps, unless challenged by a new attitude, could create habitual depressive thinking? Don't forget to check Albert Ellis and his list of Ten Irrational Beliefs that might warrant your consideration, even if such irrational beliefs once worked well for you.

Some beliefs may be unhelpful at best, and some may even be destructive of personal well-being. Others may need to be shared with trusted friends, before discarding them for those you believe will provide you with far more helpful alternate choices. Be brave – face the drainers, and find the energy gainers, and reap the benefits for others as well!

But do remember – a commitment to consciously adopting a *new* constructive behaviour will require practice, to successfully displace the old habitual thinking or old behaviour with a new and automatic response. More on this later.

Notes

1 The Conversation, 9 February 2024, by Jon Jureidini (affiliated with Critical Psychiatry Network Australasia), asking the Question, "Why are so many Australians taking anti-depressants?" He stated that one in seven in Australia are said to be prescribed anti-depressants.

2 The MBTI tool is used extensively internationally: in workplaces interested in staff/individual differences, in marriage counselling, as well as for individuals who struggle to understand why they feel so different or inadequate when compared with others. 'Gifts Differing' by Myers & Myers was written in 1980 before the assessment tools were devised.

Chapter 9

Grief and loss explored

Here we consider various forms of grief and loss, with several examples of personality factors that can prevent honest communication impacting possible resolutions. Questions of guilt, mind-reading, and inevitable emotional after-effects, both for clients and carers, may also make communications between individuals more difficult. Such problems will be more obvious when several factors or events contribute a cumulative effect to the unexplored grief. Debriefing after shared traumatic stories is essential, and often requires more than vocal communication. Imagery, using several different treatment options, is again described in applying Gestalt-based techniques. These offer powerful adjuncts to resolving grief through processing heavy undesirable memories by overlaying and replacing them with beautiful, healthy alternatives. Lastly, we reflect on how suffering itself can play a part in growing resilience while dealing with the devastation of traumas.

What picture first comes to mind that portrays personal *grief* to you? Is it some deep sadness personally experienced by you, or someone dear to you? Was that sadness related to the loss of someone or some*thing* held precious, still deeply missed? Or is that grief felt as an ongoing other feeling that still invades your thinking when you are left alone: like anger about what someone has done to you, or maybe an unresolved frustration that remains just below your emotionally controlled behaviour when around others? Maybe it is a loss of self-respect, or the loss of trust in others, something that frequently invades your thoughts, not seeming to ever go away?

Grief comes in many forms, so demands different skills.

My experience in counselling people from various walks of life has encompassed all of these issues, but fortunately not all in the same person. For some, not being conscious of what grieved them was yet to be uncovered. For others the depth of

DOI: 10.4324/9781003474746-9

feelings prior to coming into a psychologist's room or caring person's office has already been alluded to – "a grief that can't be spoken". So the challenge first and foremost is to establish a rapport that enables that unexplored sensitive subject to be revealed. I guess by now you realise that the time factor will depend on the individual, and how comfortable they are to freely share innermost thoughts and feelings with another.

The more extroverted, socially outgoing individual will often engage at a superficial level quite quickly. But, beware: the *real* person may still be hiding. Many a comedian comes to mind: very funny, entertaining, but, underneath, a deeply sensitive person wearing a mask! Even though you listen well, and the person talks a lot, you will need to bring a sensitivity that is willing to move ahead of the one sharing, letting them know that you believe their time is precious, that you want to help them identify what really brings them to seek your help. No matter how they may seem "so together", and happy to converse, it is likely that their real need will only slowly be revealed, unless of course you give the invitation. You see, often the outgoing, seemingly confident person is good at hiding their emotions, intentionally, in order to keep the sociable atmosphere pleasant: it is easier for the self as well as for the other.

On the other hand, the more introverted shy person, having finally made the appointment, may well be feeling so inadequate in disguising his or her emotions that an attempt will be made to say as little as possible. Our task as helpers is to *pace and lead*:[1] to stay with the person for as long as they need, before encouraging more communication between you. This may mean that you acknowledge your perception about the person feeling uncomfortable – affirming that such feelings are quite understandable, given that coming to speak with a stranger takes a lot of courage! Similar expressions will reveal not only a concern for them but will help to normalise their feelings. It will also assure them of your own sensitivity to their needs, which will encourage trust in their having made *you* their choice of someone to speak with.

Grief: feelings that need to be spoken

Let me share with you a couple of contrasting clients, to illustrate how grief can be experienced and shared differently. The first of these reminds us again that the presenting problem may mask other more crucial problems. The challenge then is for us to help this person discover their issue(s), so that they can clarify or *own* what really needs to be addressed.

Marlene came with an apparent anxiety problem, which bordered on what she had been told was an obsessive-compulsive disorder (OCD). She reported always having to check whether she had left lights on, the iron not unplugged, the doors left unlocked, or some combination of any of these – all of it driving her husband of almost twenty years to distraction! She hated being this way and admitted it had become worse in the last year. Background details initially suggested a contented wife, mother of two late teenage girls, and one who was quite glad to have no financial worries. Marlene claimed general contentment in her life, especially with not having to work like many of her friends!

I was not convinced that the irrational anxiety-driven behaviours could be explained by the story she gave; there had to be more. Going back to life before her marriage suddenly revealed a plainer picture: a mid-teenage pregnancy that resulted in her being sent away to have the baby and his subsequent adoption. Parental shame and her own loneliness were part of a very real grief she carried in silence.

Which do you think would be the best course of support?

Of course, needing to hear the full story is a given. However, giving her time to affirm her feelings about that event years ago was the present priority. She needed to be assured of my concern for her, with an appropriate indication of understanding how this must have been a terrible time of absolute grief, with a profound sense of isolation. Then I heard how she managed her life after that: she had returned to her rural environment some four years later, when the previous relationship which had produced her pregnancy was resumed, and they had happily married. But the son given up was, unbelievably to me, *never talked about*! It was as if she had closed the book on this incredibly sad and traumatic chapter of her life, as together they then wrote a new one. When I asked if her grief still erupted at times, her sadness became really evident, as she sobbed about what as a couple was never shared between them – the son they'd had but never known!

Marlene had no inkling of what Jeff might also have been feeling, nor was she confident to begin that conversation with him alone. Jeff was her silent rock, she explained, who rarely showed feelings though he was always quietly supportive of her and their two girls. Although he was not much of a talker, she believed he did care about her.

Faulty mind-reading creates problems and prevents healing.

The OCD symptoms were now considered less important, but encouragement was needed for Marlene to trust me with what she had shared. That trust also needed to extend to Jeff, given my insight that he also needed to become part of her grief resolution. Though diffident, she agreed to bring Jeff in for a joint session, and for me to open up the subject of their lost child. This was arranged basically on the grounds that she needed his help to overcome her fears of forgetting so many things. Jeff offered no resistance: in fact, he surprisedly indicated that he was really glad to be asked. His genuine concern quickly became evident, with the result that even in his first session with me, I was able to ask if he ever thought about the child they had given up years before. Marlene was obviously surprised about his immediate response:

"Every day! Not a day goes by without my wondering what he is doing, how he's going!"

Then Marlene spoke directly to him, saying: "But you never talk about him!"

"Neither do you, Marlene – and I got the impression it was too painful, so I'd better not!"

Amazing, really! So many people assume that they know what the important other is thinking, while being unaware of the real thoughts and feelings that remain so well hidden. After they had safely shared their sadness within my accepting environment, I knew they needed to articulate what they had separately wondered about their lost child, and to reflect openly about him now. Asking some pertinent questions meant that I was also able to present some potential future scenarios, such as that their adopted child, by then in his twenties, might already be exploring who his mother was. They were encouraged to consider such possibilities together, in order for them, and possibly eventually for their girls, to be prepared for these scenarios.

Their homework was set: to share their newly awakened grief together, but also to clarify how and what they might need to share with their girls. I carefully alerted them to possible negative reactions as well as potential positive outcomes. At that point, Marlene already seemed to have forgotten why she came!

Sharing grief that allows moving forward to positive growth

Unbelievably, only ten days later, Marlene made another appointment, which brought in a quite different woman from the one I first met. That very week, a letter from the adoption agency in their state capital had written, wondering if she was interested in the adoptee making some contact! Understandably they were quite blown away (as was I!) – in fact, both were ready to reply immediately in the affirmative.

Over the next few months, I was privileged to hear of their greatest ongoing excitement: a planned trip interstate to meet their son, having received from him a short video of his recent marriage! The young wife had encouraged his searching for his mother. I could only imagine how the additional information, finding not only his mother but his biological father as well, was received. Without a doubt, this would be an intense time for them all, with much explaining – and a great deal of emotional energy on both sides, particularly for the son to absorb his parents' story, and its impact on him personally.

The years of silent grief expressed in their initial session together with me stood in stark contrast with the content of their last: the shared grief had enabled huge excitement to be released!

That grief, previously denied and hidden, had resulted in some disturbing behaviours that needed serious attention, not least being the lack of sharing of their individual emotional needs. Surely, we also see here a wonderful example of how amazing our minds are, creating awkward situations and physical behaviours that in the end *can* result in good possible solutions, even solutions *consciously* unimagined.

By the way, the repetitive checking had disappeared within weeks – new thoughts, activities, and the resolved grief had turned her mourning into dancing! Marlene was one client who did return a number of times, but not to dwell on the past or with a need for help. Rather, she wanted to share with me her joys and her relief, having discovered many positive things her son had experienced with his adoptive family. And her girls loved finding that they had a big brother. What privileges we carers can unexpectedly participate in!

In the next example of grief and loss, I hope you will understand something of how working with people in distress may also bring heaviness for you, as you enter their circumstance and consequent emotional states. Sometimes you might even wish you'd not been told. One such person comes to mind: a young woman who was totally in grief about a failed marriage, wondering if she had done the wrong thing by taking her children away. I will spare you many of the details that disturbed me for quite some time, but the details here will be sufficient to describe how we too can experience grief and its associated feelings, if only through vicarious sharing.

Don't minimise your own grief when sharing others' grief.

Jenni had three young children whom she loved deeply, always concerned for their best interests. She first saw me when, in her concern about her husband's frequent angry outbursts towards her, she had finally found the courage to move to her parents' home some distance away. The potent effect of Bill's intractable alcoholic dependency had become the major contributor to that tough decision. This included Jenni's fear that his violent temper and bullying of her would in the end impact the children. She had herself never feared her own parents, so her lack of experience of life outside her happy contented family contributed to a mistrust about the best decision she should make. Jenni had frequently warned Bill of her intention to leave unless his awful aggressive alcoholic behaviour changed.

Occasional improvements had been made which for some months convinced her to stay, but always in trepidation that his violence would again erupt. She became less confident, and admitted she felt conflicted about leaving him. Her parents had encouraged her to take a break away from him, allowing the loss of his family and time alone to hopefully prove that his intentions to change were serious and trustworthy. Her initial visit to me sought reassurance that this move was not something which would make things worse. I listened and then some, as she vacillated between feeling relief, feeling guilt, yet also feeling remorse and sadness about the loss of the happy and safe marriage she'd originally envisaged for her family. Somehow her own diminished sense of personal confidence had largely contributed to why she now sought help.

By the end of her first visit, Jenni indicated a deep concern for her husband and for his relationship with his children from which she believed she was now excluding him. I wanted her to review these mixed feelings, gently challenging her perception that the break-up was entirely her responsibility. She agreed to another visit, and I sincerely hoped she would stay firm in her resolution to stay separated.

She did not keep the next appointment, and simply cancelled it, reporting by phone that she was doing ok; she had made regular visits back home with the youngest child, and said that Bill seemed happier that she was trying to make it work. I expressed some concern but understood that we can only be there to support and encourage, not take responsibility for choices that others make.

Some weeks later, however, another appointment in the book had me wondering what the next thing in Jenni's story might be. She came into the room with a distraught, tired face, leaving me in no doubt that something quite serious was forthcoming. Suffice to say, the emotions that poured out of her were absolute grief, punctuated by words of guilt: "How could I have let this happen? What sort of mother am I?" Slowly the truth came out. A number of day visits back to her home had gone reasonably well, leaving her feeling confident things were improving, so the end could not have been predicted. During the final visit only days ago, he had called her into their bedroom, and she went, innocently leaving her child playing happily in the kitchen. Suddenly and unexpectedly, he had pulled a gun from under the bed – her alarm bells rang so loudly that she raced out of the house, without thinking. What-to-do thoughts suddenly became totally entangled by her thoughts of what she had *done*: she had left her child with his dad, who had a gun in his hands!

She then recalled her incredible next reaction when she heard the gun fire: a swift desperate rush to get her child, fearing the worst. Her grief about her initial reaction, which had sprung automatically out of fear and self-protection, was further explored as instinctively born out of concern for the other children.

Exploring quietly *what* she had done gave her time to remember things more clearly. In hindsight she realised her immediate response *was* to the threat to her safety. Jenni had always believed Bill would never hurt the children – he loved them too much. She remembered her self-loathing, only somewhat reduced on finding her little one, sobbing but alive. She found her husband dead in the bedroom. Trauma on trauma!

I recall this session even now as tragic, unbelievably horrible, and for both of us. The potential disasters that Jenni poured out needed no promptings: she had been over these many times. They prevented her from sleep, and even now made it so difficult to focus on looking after her children. Her parents were again her place of safety and support.

Imagination: positive reflections and future focus

During this long and emotionally draining session and two subsequent sessions, Jenni was eventually able to grasp some small elements of relief. During a brief, guided imagery for relaxation, Jenni allowed herself to imagine a place of quiet, watching her children play at the beach. While she relaxed in that scene, I quietly and slowly reflected with her on three important precious prospects she now had. One was the wonder of still having all three children. The second was how grateful she was for her parents' love and supportive care. And thirdly, she was able to indicate her acceptance, with some thankfulness, that the relational struggles she had bravely endured for years were finally over and would no longer continue for her children.

How I wished I could do more! But what was finally sinking in, for Jenni too, was that her grief, her sadness, and her sense of guilt would only change with time, when she deliberately gave her focus to her children, possible as a result of the recent events, and now live without fear. Gradually a right reflection on the choices she had made would restore a personal sense of balance about *future* choices needing to be made.

What sort of reflection are you experiencing right now? You may feel deep empathy for what Jenni went through – before and after what could have been an even more incredibly difficult tragedy. Perhaps you can imagine what questions, what feelings I was left with after that session! The next person, somehow, would need my full attention, but that session was, yes, somewhat shortened, as my own personal need to debrief with a colleague became imperative.

Debriefing after shared traumas

I am sure you know for yourself what I reiterate here: *debriefing* outside the trauma room after such cases is essential! Today the SES (Fire and Flood State

Emergency Services), Police, Medical, and Paramedic services are all aware of this. Not just as good practice, but also to ensure a healthy wholeness for all individual carers who want to continue to provide best assistance to those in need. We are all human, and though some of us will be more consciously aware of what impacts on our personal lives, each of us will eventually understand the cumulative effects on us of listening to personal experiences which call us to connect at a deep level of concern.

Here it may be helpful to recall a couple of the earlier examples of grief that were written about under different topics. For example, those cases mentioned under depression (Chapter 7), like that of Harry, who, due to losing his job, experienced an enormous but unresolved real sense of grief and loss, a sense of uselessness, having grasped inadequate and inappropriate ways of dealing with that loss. And do you remember Philippa, who experienced psychotic episodes after a brain injury? Even if we've only broken a leg, or have spent time recuperating after an illness, we may catch a glimpse of how a health issue, even if only a transient illness, can impact us with a sense of grief. A permanent physical or emotional change will impact even more so. Colin, also mentioned in Chapter 7, personally suffered from the trauma and grief of war and, on top of that depression, experienced a psychologically devastating grief associated with having had his financial security bitterly taken away. This was heightened because it was inflicted on him by the very people he believed should be trustworthy – a terrible sense of betrayal, grief, and loss!

It may help for you to revisit other names from earlier chapters, to reflect on how much grief and loss was also part of their stories: the child Tom and his mother Sharon (Chapter 1), Karena (Chapter 3), Martha (Chapter 3), and Cheryl and Graham (Chapter 5), to mention just a few. Very rarely when we listen carefully do we find that it is a single issue that needs attention. It may also be a good time for you to think about each of these people, with a greater awareness of what other issues may have been addressed, perhaps even under an alternative chapter heading.

Different disguises of grief and loss are equally significant

We briefly pause to reflect again on Marion, from Chapter 8 – you may recall her grief that was not about physical loss due to illness, but more to the personal loss of her mother in earlier life. That contributed to her having less support when experiencing new demands, a loss that still held an importantly relevant impact on her, as a mother herself now feeling incapable of giving. In other words, her unexpressed grief had expanded when the reality of life's demands played out in her loss of "Me Time", something that previously had not been recognised as an essential ingredient for her sense of well-being.

Many forms of grief, mostly attended by a sense of loss, are commonly ignored or regarded as fleeting. Thankfully, our bodies can heal many of the superficial hurts we experience, and sometimes amazingly quickly. But those that are deeper, not so visible but have more of an emotional impact on us as individuals (whether on our hearts, minds, or within our spirits), these hold a greater need to be opened up, to allow healing beneath – much like the sores that form superficial scabs but which house messy, toxic fluids that need to be debrided, offering the cleansing that releases a greater healing potential.

Pictures used to effectively replace ugly memories

We have demonstrated that hidden sufferings benefit from being spoken aloud, but often this will not be enough. There may be a need to consider one of the therapeutic approaches that allow *new* images, healthier pictures to cover over those past events that haunt. I'm thinking of several people for whom such traumas had remained so vividly that the grief persisted as if the loss happened only yesterday.

One such case involved another horrific car accident, which Amanda the paramedic had attended. Though somewhat similar to Kylie's case mentioned in Chapter 5, in this incident the driver had suffered massive injuries and had died on the way to hospital. As a well-experienced "ambo" (paramedic), Amanda's reaction was to be expected – she had always known she would need a few days off. Yet some weeks later she struggled to report for work, still having nightmares. She said she felt silly about seeing me, like others who also claim, "this shouldn't be necessary for an ambo, given it is my job!"

However, it became apparent that this was not a typical reaction for her, and she needed to understand how and why this was different. I asked her to recall as much as possible about this tragedy. Her reflections recalled nothing peculiar, until one last detail, mentioned in a somewhat offhand manner. She had lately been experiencing some disturbing dreams. These concerned a much-loved aunt who had died years ago, but according to Amanda this could not be part of her problem. On further reflection, however, she did recall that the person who tragically died so recently in the accident had looked a little like an image she had of her aunt in her youth, from a photo Amanda had always loved.

When specific recalls are encouraged, it is always possible that memories that have been lost in time can suddenly erupt. Some seem to have been deliberately buried, potentially explained by how *forgetting* actually can reduce unwanted disturbing images and their associated feelings. Not surprising to me, but certainly now to Amanda, here we may see how this old memory of her aunt may have dovetailed unconsciously with a recent trauma. Current repetitive dreams of her aunt suggested that perhaps the loss of her aunt may somehow have been related to her shaken confidence in coping with work traumas. Though she prided herself on her naturally strong ability to cope with pain of all types, she now quietly shared with me that her aunt had died of a sudden stroke. For some time, her death had left Amanda with a strongly *distorted* gross picture of her loved aunt, one that belied the beautiful memory she'd previously had of her. After some years without that stressful picture of her aunt, it had now savagely returned in her dreams.

So, which of the two deaths reported on by Amanda do you think needed to be given immediate attention?

In unravelling how these two personally distressing events had become intertwined, Amanda was asked to reflect before the next session if either one of them seemed now to be the more upsetting. We completed a short time of relaxation before she left, agreeing to revisit some lovely memories she had of her aunt, experienced when on holiday with her as a child. Those warm feelings experienced then became part of the positive elements to be used in the next session. As you might expect, recalling the more personal and sleep-depriving dreams, where her aunt's disturbing death still featured in various forms, helped her resolve the question of where we would focus the therapy.

Switching: opposing pictures technique to replace unwanted memories

Because Amanda had already begun her therapy at home, recalling and writing down a list of enjoyable memories which she brought with her, I was able to use the technique of "switching" pictures as the main approach. This is another technique based on Gestalt psychology and promoted by practitioners of Neuro-Linguistic Programming (NLP).[2] This treatment option of picture switching depends on the principle that one can't hold two opposing pictures at the same time. This is particularly effective when the desired picture can overlay the undesirable one and is quickly reinforced with newly acquired positive associations.

Relaxation is often used to facilitate this procedure. Amanda comfortably slipped into her preferred relaxation mode, imagining a spot at the beach where she had spent lovely times with her aunt, and then holding that beautiful, coloured picture as a still picture on an imagined screen. She was then asked to think of a neutral picture, changing the focus for several minutes. We briefly talked about her job, what she enjoyed about it normally, with another neutral picture deliberately suggested, almost as a distraction. Then she was again asked to put the earlier positive picture of her aunt on to her full screen, calling her to notice her feelings of enjoyment. This was essential before then getting her to imagine moving that picture into one corner of her screen, to become just a tiny picture. This required regularly checking that she could actually visualise my simple verbal directions: "Can you see . . . and is it in the corner?" There was a careful checking of "Now what can you see?" after the next suggested activity to assure me that the process was working for her.

Amanda was instructed to allow her remembered picture of her aunt's deathly sad face to momentarily appear on the imagined large screen, very briefly recalling how she felt about that event, before quickly *switching* that picture to the corner of the screen, so that the now enlarged small but happy colour picture from the corner takes centre stage, swapped with the sad one, now vastly reduced in size and importantly reduced to only black and white, into the corner. With the large colourful screen now visible, some moments of reflection enabled Amanda to fully access her relaxed state. She came to appreciate that each time the beautiful picture of her aunt was briefly interrupted by her recalling of her sadly distorted face, it was dismissed as quickly as possible. The word "switch" or "change" became the instruction that was used a number of times as a simple procedure, with a few minutes of relaxed neutral reflections before doing the same process over again. It is important to note that after each repetition, it was necessary to check how Amanda was feeling about the sad distorted face of her aunt and how readily diminished the clarity of that picture had become, to ascertain the effectiveness of the switching method to modify her negative feelings.

Are you a bit sceptical about how and why this works? Do some research. Perhaps you could reflect about what happens when you yourself have felt disturbed by a cinema film. What plays out afterwards can depend on many elements that you may not always be conscious of. For example, if you have been in a good mood beforehand, you will feel quite differently about the film than if you went to it already feeling despondent. If you also include a prior personal experience, regardless of whether positive or negative, the feelings you leave the theatre with may be even more exaggerated. Of course, most people almost instinctively grasp the need to do something to offset that powerful cinematic experience – either to nullify its negative effect, or, if it's been positive, to keep that emotional high going. The café next door does well! Challenging the unacceptable feelings is provided by means of an alternative focus. Simply telling oneself *not* to think about something is mostly unhelpful, so that an effective resolution requires you to choose to put something else in its place.

So it is with memories: ones that are beautiful we usually choose to hang on to. Those that are disturbing, however, at critical times still do demand our attention. Some people try hard to forget. Some experience an involuntary mental shutdown. By fighting memories which have caused the trauma, like taking on a new busy schedule of activities, some sufferers can avoid additional stress. Some find relief by grappling to understand the circumstances of the trauma; this can also provide an adjunct to again living victoriously over the intensity of the trauma and its impact, with revitalising enjoyment.

Suffering is minimised by moving beyond debilitating grief and loss.

Recently I was privileged to engage with a new arrival in Australia, a refugee fleeing religious persecution, and had been refused entry after trying to enter illegally.[3] Her husband had three weeks earlier been allowed in, just prior to the laws imposed that made her case for asylum in Australia so much less possible. Ten years on, that is still her situation!

We'll call her Nellie, with an aside here that though we may have roles as carers, mentors, psychologists, and in various other professions, so often we are called on to just be friends. We are fellow humans on a journey, and because we are caring people, our fellow travellers will share their specific struggles with us. We quite naturally listen well, so we also lend a supportive hand! But as we enter their suffering, share their grief, we find we also gain from these interactions, including a growth in understanding our own humanity.

Friendships – fellow travellers

The truth in the words of Christ which affirm "it is more blessed to give than to receive" has been affirmed again in the friendship with this brave young woman. Her traumas involved many different elements while being forced to survive within an island incarceration. This had lasted for over six long years – involving medical care, many court cases, and determined carers – before she was finally granted permission to join her husband, but as an illegal migrant, with no financial support available for her future here. Mind-blowing really! Hard to understand, let alone really be able to deeply share her emotions. Yet the sharing of her experiences provides insights into the very resilience that one human can develop, in spite of the gross suffering and incredible grief and loss imposed through politically determined abuse.

Nellie reported how she had gradually developed personal strategies, learned through countless experiences she had to pass through in order to do more than survive. These included inspiring herself by personal reflections around nature; memories of home that remained clear; and keeping to herself, to prevent the awful sharing that occurred between other helpless but more angry victims. During her aloneness, she experienced a spiritual awareness of a far bigger picture, finding and reconnecting with a liberating faith in her Creator, one she had innocently enjoyed as a child. Such contemplative practice regularly, though intermittently, was able to lift her out of her language-deprived, socially impossible situation, despite there being little hope of her ever changing her living conditions. Along with her practice of meditation in nature, her unbearable isolation was only relieved by occasional brief phone connections with her husband, and brief mobile phone interchanges with parents left behind.

Resilience through suffering

During her rugged time of survival, Nellie learned to discern those few people who could be trusted and those who could not: only possible through quiet reflection, contemplation of her very self, as well as those around her. She made some positive decisions too: deliberately choosing to refrain from fighting the present ugliness with anger and soul-destroying negativity.

Nellie also had to learn new ways of living that released her from her isolation: one way was to find someone less able, less fortunate than herself. Having acknowledged her understandable self-focus, she began to attempt to think beyond herself. While trying to understand her own complex self, she also became more aware that others may not understand themselves or why they do what they do. She discovered that in recognising her own weaknesses, she became less critical of others. She reports learning humility, even in having to admit a need for help – she who had come from so much. She rediscovered many biblical truths that taught her to love others: finding a needy stray animal grew her capacity to love, and then to receive love. This too was part of her maturing through years of suffering; such a maturity now enables her to be a blessing to others, in spite of still struggling within the reality of her own grief and loss. Understandably, this great sadness still frequently breaks into her consciousness, with a future that is still very unpredictable.

REFLECTIVE EXERCISES

- Has this last case in particular reminded you of some of the great people of the past you've read about and admired? We could expect many of them suffered from some form of depression. Yet such people, through great hardship, gained important personal insights. They *attained greater understanding* about those perpetrators of evil against them, recorded so that we who have not suffered may also vicariously learn from these. You may have personal experiences to support this perspective. Human character is often developed because of trauma, not simply in spite of it.
- Maybe re-read some of the stories of human survival that are often quite amazing: Joan of Arc, Martin Luther King, Nelson Mandela. Another

example is Viktor Frankl, who after his release from his internment in Auschwitz wrote his psychological memoir. His book *Man's Search for Meaning* became a tribute to how he survived. It contains so many wise insights that a thorough read is warranted. One such truth may encourage your search: his understanding that there is one thing that *can't* be taken from humans – "to choose one's attitude in any given circumstance".

- As we read how others have survived such events, ask yourself what you see as their greatest resource: beliefs about a future time or place when released? Or was there a solid trust in terms of their faith journey, knowing they were not alone, that enabled their present endurance? The challenge we are left with is to seek a greater understanding of resilience, it being the really powerful aspect of suffering that we'd prefer not to personally experience!
- Reconsider what a grief that can't be spoken really means to you. How do you feel about talking with others who perhaps can't find the words? Perhaps you may dare to suggest alternative means of sharing: painting, writing, or music. Or you may be good at telling an allegorical or fictional story that might speak to the feelings which can't be named yet will gently reveal and validate those feelings. Used sensitively, any of these can be such great tools when there are no adequate words.
- Reflect on some of your friends who want your friendship, not your counsel: how do you demonstrate that you care? Have you become more conscious of times when you are not comfortable in dealing with their pain? So that you better cope, have you developed alternative responses to using your previous distractions that might have suggested you don't really care?
- Consider those who have shared their stories of grief, their pain, their unexpected and unjust circumstances still raw to them. Do they perhaps challenge us as carers to form better ways of enabling *others* to develop good strategies that can bring about wholeness?
- Do you feel inspired to develop new skills that might help others *overcome* or *better manage* those more difficult circumstances? Your psychological helper toolbox needs to include those various tools that bring about personal growth, providing potential opportunities that might enable the sufferer to benefit, as well as those around them.
- You will have your own examples of people who have suffered much but who have more than survived. Triumphed! In this chapter with its focus on grief and loss, I hope you grasp again the wonderful privilege

to walk alongside those who experience pain and suffering, despite being a costly and time-consuming commitment. This will be true regardless of whether that grief or loss is physical or mental, emotional or spiritual, learning from them even as you offer a helping hand.

I do hope that some of the examples I've recorded here will also affirm an old truism: a shared sorrow can diminish the suffering, while a shared joy will increase it!

Notes

1 This is an Ericksonian technique that is really invaluable with more challenging individuals.

2 It is acknowledged that NLP is generally regarded as pseudo-scientific in regard to core assumptions about the way that there are connections between neurological processes (*neuro-*), language (*linguistic*), and acquired behavioural patterns (look at Wikipedia on NLP for details). While promoted by NLP practitioners, the effectiveness of the switching technique can itself be adequately explained and validated in terms of both Gestalt Therapy and Cognitive Behavioural Therapy.

3 She has given permission for me to recount part of her experience, anonymised. Though she is reunited with her husband, many external factors remain unresolved; she still has no rights to work, study, or look towards citizenship in Australia.

Chapter 10

Mental illness, health and wellbeing

The various sub-headings within this chapter indicate a range of issues about mental health that are of benefit to identify and understand in regard to diagnosis and support. The overall understanding, far from comprehensive, is broadly based, encouraging the reader to consider associated attitudes and beliefs about what mental illness may or may not really be. The chapter moves between behaviours that are misunderstood, being unusual or different (exhibited by those on the outer spectrum of individual differences), to the inclusion of others that warrant serious intervention. Historical attitudes are presented before questions are asked that revolve around how best to manage people exhibiting problem behaviours, particularly as a result of taking illicit drugs. We also try to encourage an openness about how to understand the complexity that undergirds any evidence of mental dysfunction, some of which all people may experience, though for differing periods of time. Misdiagnosis is also noted, as this can inevitably contribute to lasting problems that may well have been avoided with more awareness of the basis of the inception of the presenting problem.

The preceding five chapters (Chapters 5–9) have tried to tease out the many and varied problems that demand help from a caring outsider, and for which we maintain that listening is not enough. Deliberately, it is only now that we have included this chapter on Mental Illness, purposefully after a greater exploration of commonly experienced problems that are not necessarily health issues deemed to be mental *illness*.

But on reading the last chapter, you may wonder at what point it becomes necessary to consider when behaviour has become so abnormal that "mental illness" needs to be contemplated. This is an important and complex question that deserves a rather large solitary chapter. There is also confusion with the terms "mental illness", "well-being" and "mental health", often indiscriminately used interchangeably. During this chapter we attempt to provide case examples that demonstrate greater clarity about what each means, and where they may be best used.

DOI: 10.4324/9781003474746-10

However, it is important to first note that we humans often feel uncomfortable with people we don't understand. Perhaps out of fear, some may even assume that unusual, "different" people need to be challenged, even forcibly changed, or worse still, removed from society. We might even go so far as to describe a person whose behaviour is off the "normal" scale as being "completely insane". Though the general word used historically for mental illness included these words, "insane" has become a word with quite different connotations, either as a pejorative or at times currently even used as a *positive* term of flattery!

I would suggest that today we like to censure any word that looks like an unkind descriptor, to find another that is more acceptable, and one that fits into a politically correct world. It is important that words such as mental illness are well defined and understood, and when used correctly are of benefit for health and well-being. Cynically speaking, using the "right" word can also justify some financial support being granted, which might encourage the recipient to keep that descriptor alive, rather than contemplate becoming well! Here is yet another potential instance of secondary gain.

Historical attitudes to mental illness

Some of us may recall hearing of or indeed may have personal family stories, about people in the past who were admitted to psychiatric institutions, because certain behaviours meant that such people were deemed unfit for society. We are horrified about decisions by the "experts" who identified certain individuals as insane: for example, women suffering serious postnatal childbirth delusions or extreme menopausal symptoms, who were involuntarily incarcerated, and some indeed never released.[1]

Today we are also more aware of the cruelty of *past* attitudes towards gay or lesbian people, whose dispositions, values and beliefs were kept hidden, simply to avoid criminal charges. Clearly, being different is not *of itself* a mental illness issue, though it severely impacts many people's mental health because of it. Rejecting differences of any kind is explained by some as inherent in the natural human inclination to tribalism associated with primal human needs of identity and belonging further explored in Chapter 14. For example, we see many thinking Australians disturbed and challenged by the slow-moving tide that confronts the inhumane treatment of first-nation people, so treated because they were seen as different, physically and culturally! They are still struggling to be acknowledged and respected by some of the descendants of "white" Australian colonial invaders of the past. Not only is this a national problem, but a worldwide issue seen for example in "Black lives matter".

Universally, we are charged with a need for greater understanding of our differences. This includes our many ways of viewing "normality", and this can seriously challenge the broad spectrum of individual differences that makes labelling so difficult. However, labelling still occurs – and often with the best of intentions: to help us find best options for helping someone whose behaviour is problematic. Unfortunately, by doing so, often those with different labels from our own can be treated as people to be feared, or kept at a distance, since, for many, being different poses a threat. Even when understood and carefully explained in terms of their being different, many people still simply question their own perspective of what is normal, not least in relation to what is acceptable. This unease leaves many without satisfying answers as to how to resolve their conflicted internal view of self *and* of others they are so different from.

Understanding our differences and respecting those who are "different" does not mean that we simply accept all behaviours. But it does pose a conundrum about what to do with people who break our societal laws, particularly those who behave in ways that tragically impact adversely on others. Locking them up and throwing away the key, however, is not a response that demonstrates a belief in "loving others as we love ourselves". We all know the phrase "there but for the grace of God go I", traditionally attributed to the mid-16th-century compassionate and humble man, John Bradford. His distress when sorrowfully watching a group of "criminals" being led to execution suggests that, even then, not all people thought criminals needed to be excluded permanently from society, even if just for its protection. But surely, a solution should be found that would be considered an appropriately humane one.

I'm reminded of our using many second-hand building materials while building our mudbrick home. We procured some large solid timber doors that some 70 plus years prior had been part of a mental health facility, then called an asylum. (Interesting use of the word, is it not? A place of safety, protection, refuge for healing, and a concept still abused in relation to how some treat asylum seekers today.) The doors were covered with many coats of paint which we sandblasted back to their original beautiful wood. We then discovered why they were so heavy: embedded with thick steel plates to make it impossible for mentally disturbed inmates, male or female, to break out from! Such was the consequent restraining power at the time given to those suffering mental illness, and often considered incurable.

Reasonable approaches to mental illness

This historical picture demonstrates one far-reaching consequence of the general term "mental illness", and sadly, the term still conjures up many unresolved social issues. The first one relates to the question of personal responsibility expected of an individual should they be labelled with a mental illness. For example, it seems that even our legal system in Australia today is increasingly caught up with conceding leniency on the ground of mental illness, a common practice observed that finds vindication for certain crimes committed. A second issue we are confronted with relates to the impact on the *individual*, whose label permanently judges that person with the associated illness and is one that cannot easily be challenged or rescinded. This often generates a negative self-belief that seriously reduces the person's potential for independent living.

In a school setting, a more positive option of support for a child diagnosed with a mental illness as a result, for example, of an acquired brain injury (ABI) in Australia today is that funding is readily available for that child. But sadly this often means that for another child whose disability is deemed minor or low-key but equally disabling, such as having been born with a limited brain capacity in a specific area, government funding is almost impossible to find. Having a specific learning difficulty, for example, or a hearing loss, may result in a child being considered as less than deserving of funding and even of a teacher's interest, particularly if no untoward negative behaviour is evident. There are also serious challenges in deciding what specific behaviours to modify when giving help to people exhibiting a mental illness, let alone *how* this action can ethically be defensible.

The idea that behaviour is formed from our cognitive processes always remains pertinent to the discussion of mental illness. The word "mental" itself implies brain activity which at least allows for some cerebral outworking of the mind. Sometimes, however, "normal" individuals may evidence little rational cognition or conscious thinking, particularly apparent when we consider some of their choices of action. Take for example someone who readily eats the rest of that block of chocolate, just because it is there: only afterwards may they think how stupid that was, and then ask "why did I do that?".

Reflection: Can you think about some personal examples that happen spontaneously, but which you might later regret?

You may find it easy to relate to a more serious example: imagine, at the beginning of the day, you are late for work, when another objectionable driver cuts into the busy city-bound traffic, preventing you the careful driver from getting through that orange light . . . road rage comes to the surface … boiling now . . . And if our questionable, sudden anger were to result in an accident, is it right to assume that *any normal* person would find legitimate excuses? Surely, the mind was unable to function *normally* on the basis of stress, lack of sleep, or had too much alcohol, drug addiction, a debilitating headache – all possible explanations that imply that the unusual, unacceptable behaviour couldn't be helped! Such a person is thus deemed not culpable, due to reduced capacity to be held responsible.[2]

Do we all have choices?

A diagnosed mental illness raises the question as to how much choice such labelled individuals realistically may have. I am reminded of one adult male client whose schizophrenia was medically managed by a treating psychiatrist, but who was referred on for psychological assistance, to learn effective ways to manage his anxieties. Some progress was noted by Jimmy becoming more personally responsible: for example, taking charge of regularly keeping his appointments, though he still lived with his parents. But one night he surprisedly called at 3 a.m., to report on his latest anxiety attack. But when it was pointed out what time of night he was phoning (and this was at a time before mobile phones), he simply replied: "Oh, it's ok, I didn't wake anyone. I went down the street to phone you!" Choices – though not always well thought through!

Regardless of where we might like to draw an arbitrary line, trying to explain why we sometimes do what we do, mostly our choice of behaviours remains consistent over time – unless, of course, something mediates or facilitates an unexpected or unpredictable need to react without thinking. This is where a discerning counsellor is convinced that an appropriate intervention may enable an individual to make some thoughtful changes.

But you may have heard the old joke that asks "how many hands are needed to change a lightbulb?" – from the psychologist's perspective, it only requires the bulb to be willing! Glance back at the example given about Sabina and her car accident (Chapter 6) – note her willingness to accept being unwell, choosing the secondary gain option instead. So it seems that having the will to change a behaviour does not simply guarantee that making changes will be possible or be enduring, but it *is* an essential starting point. Clearly, a precondition to change is to want to change, to be willing to change. But then, an individual needs some hope: to have some sense of self-efficacy.

Change importantly depends on motivation.

Early in the book, we referred to the importance of our motivations. Money may well have been Sabina's motivation. But I'm also reminded of a guy who suddenly made an appointment, saying he wanted to be well. He freely volunteered his story: drugs, a marriage when he was quite young that had soon collapsed, leaving him with a young son whom now, ten years later, he wanted to see more frequently. But Peter had to get himself sorted if this could become a possibility. He seemed motivated, though several issues clearly needed to be aired to clarify what had driven him to regular use of marijuana. His drug dependency had finally not only caused him to pull out of a TAFE course (a training college), but also left him with a limited capacity to remain employed for anything more than a few weeks at a time.

Therapy involved reconsidering several long-held irrational beliefs Peter had accepted about himself – no one likes me, no one thinks I am clever, my parents will never forgive my stupid mistakes – and there were many more self-deprecating beliefs that kept him from being a well person. He now indicated he was determined to live without recreational drugs. He openly disclosed that before attending counselling, he had already spent time in a psychiatric facility, suffering from several drug-induced psychotic episodes. Peter had been prescribed anti-psychotic medication, which he resented since this meant his often being "treated as a mental case". Part of his therapy, however, involved helping him stay committed to some medication, until he proved he could achieve a stability that suggested he could do without it.

At the time of seeking psychological help, Peter was mostly sleeping in his car. You can see how therapy also involved considering other issues: encouragement to find appropriate accommodation, and to orient him to find and access some non-stressful work that he could manage. Regular sessions were essential to ensure he was making some progress, realistically maintaining his new self-confidence, and without the grandiose ideas which often co-exist with the drug use that previously had been a major part of his downfall.

Long-term effect of therapy

Check-ups over the next year hinted at great promise: Peter was on the way to being a "normal", mentally well guy. Then being off all medication, he was able to form and maintain a good relationship with his son, and also had returned and completed the study he had commenced some years before. However, he later informed me that he'd met up with some of his old druggie friends, ostensibly to help them. He was warned that this was a dangerous move, with the potential risk of being dragged back into their lifestyle. But sadly, he chose to ignore this warning, and the predictable happened. Peter suffered several more psychotic episodes, despite his good intentions. His future was not doomed, but now, many years later, how well he continued to live by his earlier wiser choices is not known.

There is evidence to support an understanding that drugs may induce mental states that remain for a long time in the individual's mind, affecting available choices through their distortion of thought processes. This is particularly problematic for vulnerable young minds whose brains are still forming. We cannot be sure of who will respond so negatively to drug-induced mind-control activities, but there is clear research now showing that the effect of certain drugs can remain for many months if not years. It has been reassuring, however, to find that when recreational drugs are dismissed from their day-to-day lives, people who remain committed to abstinence are more likely to return to a normal life, not suffering serious after-effects, except from those very consequences of previous behaviours while under the influence of drugs.

Similarly, if we think about prisons, for example, the consequences of past behaviours, as well as their incarceration experiences, are so difficult to completely overcome, especially when family disconnections and financial constraints are involved. We know there are some who make the most of that time, learn from their experiences and re-evaluate their past lives, and so become people with a different potential. There are others, however, who regard prison as a training opportunity for becoming better criminals, so that prison *recidivism* becomes the normal expectation.

In the same way, we cannot *assume* that all who struggle with mental health issues, even given the best opportunities available for regaining a sense of well-being, will ever be completely well. Sometimes the depth and type of mental illness precludes this phenomenon. Donna (Chapter 8) is but one example of how this recovery conjecture can be unpredictable. But there is a need to remain open, curious, and well-informed about our options to support individuals with mental health problems, and to have realistic expectations about outcomes.

Remain open to new learnings about people.

Individual differences are innumerable, so we should not give up learning alternate ways to reach out to some of these "different" people. I remember reading one account told by Milton Erickson,[3] the famous psychiatrist and psychologist who on visiting a group of psychiatric patients was told to be quiet, and not to expect a particular man to talk. He had suffered from a long-term mental illness which isolated him from all. In response, Erickson had walked over to the man and stood on his foot. The patient immediately responded by shouting: "Why did you do that?!!" Erickson was always exploring unexpected ways that might enable him to release people from their predicted mental illness restraints.

Working in cooperation with a psychiatrist over some years was interesting, providing different points of view that widened our own perspectives. This colleague specialised in psychopharmacology, and often referred people on for psychological assistance, like relaxation training, and CBT in changing beliefs, attitudes, and their respective behaviours – these not being part of his own more biologically oriented tool kit. He had come to the conclusion that for many experiencing a psychotic illness, evidenced with delusions that had developed early in life, the condition was most often, but not exclusively, associated with teenage drug-taking. More recent knowledge has enabled us to understand this conclusion: research into the effects of drugs taken by those whose brains are still developing provides a crucial insight when looking at any resultant illness.

When we gather information about people referred to us that suggest various possible forms of mental unwellness, before accepting such referrals we need to be warned; much wisdom and patience is needed, and a proper assessment of our own capacity to assist such people back into some form of normal living. We will also need to become aware of whether good social supports are readily available to them. This may involve being prepared to spend time engaging appropriately skilled external people. It will also require an understanding of the individual's own history as well as potentially that of the family, if we expect to make any breakthroughs.

Drugs and mental illness

I recall one young guy who demonstrates much of this last paragraph. Michael was finally given an ultimatum by his parents: either get counselling or move out of home. He was 26 years old, and his girlfriend had joined him in living with his parents, since he could no longer afford to rent. His mother really felt for her much-changed son, wanting him to be well. She had recently discovered drugs in his room, however, and though he claimed he was not using them anymore, she was concerned about his increasingly erratic behaviours.

His mother visited me first, to explain her reasons for her concern for her son. Michael had recently lost his job, and his girlfriend only had part-time work. He frequently borrowed money to keep his car in petrol, which he said he needed for work options. Even after getting another job, money was always inadequate. Michael was rarely home for mealtimes, so his mother had stopped keeping meals for the couple. Unlike the curious bright boy he had been as a child, Michael was reportedly either lethargic or, alternately, now often aggressive; his parents were increasingly nervous about what he would do next, and actually feared having to ask him to leave.

It seemed Michael was intent on complying with their conditional arrangement, however, having agreed to keep the appointment with me made by his mother, ostensibly to talk about his mood changes. He claimed he wanted to get help, as he finally admitted to me that he could no longer afford the drugs of choice he was addicted to. He owned up to experiencing various delusional episodes, during which he confessed to having been violent with both his father and then also his girlfriend, who subsequently had moved out. He agreed to seek medical alternatives before going on with counselling.

His follow-up appointment indicated good intentions: he had seen a doctor who had put him on methadone. Michael claimed he was already seeing some benefits: reportedly not so moody, more able to get to work on time, and fewer arguments with his parents. He regularly attended fortnightly over several months, made possible because his mother had agreed to pay the bills, including the petrol for the two-hour round trip to get psychological help! He continued to report positively each session, always giving the impression he was making great headway. After those five or more sessions, however, his mother phoned, wanting my assurance that Michael was off drugs, and continuing to make progress.

Confidentiality

Can you see the dilemma? How to be honest without breaking any confidences! I was able to ask her how *she* thought he was going, and a different story unfolded. Not only was he still exceedingly difficult to manage, but both parents had become increasingly concerned about his not working, his sleeping a lot of the day, followed by going out late at night. She also volunteered a real concern about their inability to gain from him any indications about his "wellness".

I could only say to her that from what she had told me, she had her own evidence about where Michael was at. Being careful not to divulge the client's information, I did suggest that they as parents might need to engage some outside assistance when confronting him with his apparent abuse of their kindness, with some clarity needed about whether they should still provide his accommodation. It became clear to her that their willingness to financially support him was only further facilitating his current behaviours, rather than fostering a requirement to reform his attitudes and actions. It was also fortuitous that Michael had not made another appointment, having claimed he didn't need any more help. Michael's mental "health" was determined largely by his drug dependence, with the result that his unwillingness to own that problem finally led to his mentally unhealthy state of mind that his parents also needed to face. Dishonesty is so much typically a part of addiction, and an addiction can only be overcome when deception is owned and then rejected.

Discerning the truth – confirmation from others

You may have reflected on several issues that revolve around certain beliefs commonly held about mental illness. One, clearly accepted by Michael's parents, was seen in their commitment to care for their son, initially believing he couldn't help himself. Their home was certainly a place of safety, but it actually *enabled* his mental illness through their unquestioned financial support. It had also blocked their ability to see the truth he denied. His mental status for a long time had excused his lie-telling, his belligerent treatment of others, with no concern for his parents' welfare. Ultimately, they faced the situation, resolving that it could not continue. This resulted in Michael having to be cared for by the state: without a home, no real friends, and no means of supporting himself. His determination to live on his own terms became his undoing, to his parents' incredibly great sorrow.

So you ask: was he suffering from a mental illness? Should he simply be treated as one of the many who carry the same blight of drug-dependency, without any expectation that he should be forced to take action that would restore his sense of responsibility for his choices of action? Such questions need to be confronted by us all. Equally important, this concern is relevant for lawyers, and for politically astute lawmakers and community leaders who want our society to be safer than it is, yet understandably refuse to go back to a time when such people were locked away, punished rather than rehabilitated.

So today, what is our *individual* responsibility, as a people who maintain a commitment to helping those needing and wanting our help? What factors need to be considered when supporting someone with mental health issues, and more so when potentially using drugs?

Personal vulnerability

In accepting our own limitations, we also need to be aware that without checks on our perceptions, we can be caught out by our reliance on the apparent honesty maintained by those claiming to be working towards becoming well. We need to be willing to refuse to be duped by some who simply play the game required that has made it impossible for those caring for them to become aware of the truth.

We may also need to be prepared to stop accepting those clients who are just "using us", and those supporting them financially. You will remember Sabina's dishonesty mentioned in Chapter 6, and my need to discontinue therapy on account of her dishonest bid for financial remunerations. Many other examples abound (like Ray, back in Chapter 1, with his unfounded claims for compensation) after discerning the untruth about client claims – these all re-emphasise the importance of our own integrity when helping people.

Another client where untruths come to mind is one woman whose husband was regularly seeing our psychiatrist colleague. This psychiatrist had believed the husband was doing well, with alcohol dependency no longer a problem. So he was most surprised on hearing the wife's story: alcohol was still in fact a huge problem for her husband, hence her attending for counselling to consider her future. How easily we may be hoodwinked!

In contrast to the Peters and Michaels mentioned, however, I do remember a young lady who sought help after one psychotic episode, having indulged in a group event with drugs. Sheryll was so overwhelmed by the enormous "crazy" repercussions she'd experienced as a result of drug taking, that she determined she would *never* experiment with them again! She was also determined to do whatever it took, including regular counselling over some months, to make sure she could maintain that commitment. Prior to her psychology appointment, she had been hospitalised and diagnosed as psychotic; her parents had expressed fears for her future health and well-being, deeply concerned that Sheryll had dropped out of her university course.

Sheryll was open and honest, keen to know why she was so badly affected, wanting to understand the truth about herself. Over several sessions she became more cognisant of her personality, having a strong imaginative component which I believe had made her particularly susceptible to the influences of drugs, and quite different from the friends involved with drugs who could be so convincing. We'll look at this more deeply in Chapter 14. But with such a positive insight into her beautiful creative persona more fully appreciated, she eventually came to really accept herself. She no longer felt she had to be like all the others – she could actually enjoy being who she was, unafraid to be different, even unique! Her well-being restored, now uninhibited about her own lifestyle choices and friendship opportunities, Sheryll gradually gained confidence to make her own more introverted way, no longer needing others' approval. These elements all became part of the therapy that enabled her to become a strong and mentally healthy young woman, without regrets for the potential misdemeanours made by the less well-informed others she had previously depended on and had called friends.

Mental health or mental illness

It may be helpful at this stage to ponder why I included Donna in Chapter 8 on depression, rather than in this one, with its focus on mental illness.

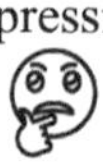 Do you have any rationale that might explain this? What implication does mental illness have for you?

It is important that we understand this whole area of mental health, though it is frequently alluded to as synonymous with mental illness. When as a young psychologist I was confronted with mental illness, there always seemed an element of fear associated with seeing such a person, as if, somehow, they would not be at all reasonable – therefore reasoning with them would be impossible. With time and experience, however, it became clearer to me that we all have aspects of oddness that might be considered irrational and unpredictable.

One important truth also became relevant in overcoming my own fear – observing someone suffering from a mental health issue demonstrated a predictability about certain behaviours that we can trust. For example, if one suffers from OCD, obsessive compulsions may be entertained on all fronts – no surprise there. Unless the diagnosis is not quite right! Thus, for example, a person may *not* really be suffering from a mental illness, but s/he may simply be expressing an individual difference, part of their DNA that may demonstrate a familial trait, or simply a familial behaviour innocently adopted as normal.

As a humorous aside, you may appreciate this true experience shared with me by a medical doctor. On seeing a patient whose injuries from a car accident were being assessed and treated, she was on the point of explaining to the patient that his crossed eyes, which sometimes occur with such a trauma, would right themselves in time – when suddenly the patient's two siblings came into the surgery, and they too each had similarly crossed eyes. The explanation would not have gone down well! But seriously, when a diagnosis of any physical or *mental* state fails to consider alternative insights, the discerned problem so labelled may stick unnecessarily for a long time and provide little assistance towards wellness.

If we go back to thinking about an OCD or "autistic" or "on the spectrum" label, such a person may demonstrate excessive concern for getting the facts right (say in relation to finances, or numbers in general), and an accuracy of reporting details is always held to be exceedingly important to them. But this does not imply a mental illness, even when it dominates that person's behaviours on many fronts. It may simply be as a result of certain values having been taken on board as all-important, essential even. Or it may just indicate a need to be consistent with their individual personality profile: someone more concerned with accurate *facts* than with feelings of empathy or with a need to understand people.

Let's briefly again consider Donna and why I had earlier chaptered her under depression. What can be learned about her state of mind when it is separated from a diagnosis of mental illness?

Today, we live in a time when depression is exceptionally prevalent; it is not only regarded as worthy of treatment, mostly without stigma, but is almost counted as normal, what normal people experience. Unfortunately however, and from my perspective and others, naming depression as a mental *illness* can itself create a problem. For example, some health insurers now refuse responsibility for certain health issues that are regarded as mental illness, and for some that even includes depression. I have counselled people who regret having ever acknowledged feeling so depressed that they had sought psychological help. This was not because the help given was unhelpful, but because when it was admitted to, their ability to get funding was refused – for a mortgage, for example, or when their health benefit refused to cover them for additional coverage, since they were deemed to have suffered from a mental illness. Yet such depression is acknowledged as being experienced most often due to an *exogenous* cause (Chapter 6), and therefore may only last for a comparatively brief episode in a person's life.

Back to the label of "psychotic" in Donna's case. This relates to her strongly felt negative thoughts that had extensively trained those around her to treat her as a "mental case", and this factor may have seriously impacted her capacity to be "normal". Clearly, she had suffered much in her mind, and a lack of understanding may have "pushed her over the edge" to make normality seem unattainable.

Misdiagnosis inevitably creates problems.

We are aware today that labelling may be useful in order to appropriately deal with or support a person experiencing certain unhelpful thoughts and their commensurate behaviours. But that labelling is often known to be detrimental to the individual, particularly if it assumes that it *perfectly* describes that person, and its truthfulness will remain *forever*. This can create an assumption that one can expect little change, unless controlled by medication. Labels can as such be devastatingly disempowering.

As I write, a news item reported an unhappy person who, during COVID, had sought and gained a phone consultation, and, without being seen, was given a script for Ritalin to deal with her apparent ADHD diagnosis. Her troubling saga unfolded over the next two years, with the wrong diagnosis meaning that the client had suffered from extraordinary drug-induced psychiatric experiences that may not have been encountered with a more appropriate diagnosis.[4]

I hope this concern will encourage you to reconsider what *your* attitude is when describing a person with a label, even if it gives a reasonably accurate picture of sorts at the time. And in fairness to any individual suffering from difficult symptoms – including someone with a serious history of a mental illness – this should not mean that we then make assumptions about the person that prevents a positive move forward.

Try to form a good habit in speaking about the sufferer, always with compassion, making sure you describe the *problem*: thoughts/beliefs/debilitating behaviours and self-doubts, or even schizophrenic ideas that the person suffers from, *rather than* that they are a schizophrenic, a social misfit, or a psychotic. Think about the term *leper* that used to label the person, but who is better described as suffering from *leprosy*!

Again, consider a person, like Marlene in Chapter 9, who had developed an unacceptable or strange set of behaviours because of an unmet need. In the same way, we may observe why one individual's need is to be *extra* careful about certain things important to them – perhaps is related to suffering the repercussions of a negative experience or lack of care, or simply a survival reaction to an unexpected and disastrous event.

I'm reminded of a young adult male who attended his first session with his mother, admitting to suffering from a diagnosed OCD mental illness, and in his case related to obsessional behaviours around hygiene and cleanliness. Together they had struggled to find the relief that would offer both comfort and some practical way forward.

Tim had always been an imaginative person, even as a small child. This seemed to have morphed into his becoming increasingly preoccupied with showering and hand washing, which inevitably made life very difficult for the rest of the family. I guess you can imagine the exaggerated frustrations when, as a teen, he had literally taken hours each day in the bathroom. He was now in early twenties, and all but his mother had lost patience with him; other family members simply accepted that his mental illness meant nothing would ever change, so they needed to make alternative arrangements for themselves.

His mother still lived in hope. After that first session, Tim agreed to come alone, to look at better ways for him to learn to *manage* his thoughts, rather than, as routinely until then, expecting others to simply make allowances for his illness. Challenging the irrational thoughts began that process. Getting him to think about how others saw his irrationally based attitudes to cleanliness was interesting to encourage though difficult for him to imagine!

The time eventually arrived when he felt safe enough to engage in imaginative relaxation, which often included imagining playing with water, though clearly outside the hygiene context. During the periods of structured relaxation, interwoven with positive enjoyment experienced with water, it became possible for Tim to reflect on "normal" hygiene behaviours. This also included seeing how his brother and sister looked on with disapproval, allowing his imagination to register those reactions as being unsatisfying for himself as well as for them.

While relaxed and contemplative, Tim was encouraged to imagine back to a time when such feelings about cleanliness had not been a problem. He then clearly described the *forgotten* picture of himself: a happy almost four-year-old, playing outside on his own in his parents' garden, naked. He remembered this as being so enjoyable. Nothing seemed to worry him then. He adored finding butterflies, caterpillars, picking flowers and making daisy chains. Then his face changed. I asked what he saw. He suddenly spoke in a subdued voice, describing the picture of some old friends of his parents arriving, the female person suddenly frowning angrily at him, telling him to "go and get some clothes on, you dirty little boy!". He remembered briefly wondering why she was so angry. But now, he remembered that very incident as being the start of his need to always be a clean boy! Without conscious awareness, this need had escalated with time. Yet he had never told his mother what he'd heard that day – indeed, until that therapy session, he had not been aware of what was behind his obsession, having completely forgotten or driven that event into conscious oblivion.

The label doesn't always explain the behaviour!

I hope you can see how important it is to encourage a person who believes they need to change some inappropriate behaviour to take time to reflect: to ask when it commenced, and what in hindsight seemed to have aroused such a reaction. But remember not to ask why! The clearer the reflection, the more likely it will be that a positive understanding be exposed that may powerfully contradict the prior behavioural choice. After all, that early commitment was not usually made with a clear and conscious rationale, or with a fundamental understanding of what had happened – so that *apparent* reactive belief could not be right or beneficial.

You will know of the many examples of children who were not only physically or emotionally abused but told *why* they were abused. On top of those heavy lies, they were usually warned never to tell anyone, or else! Only later are they able to explain why they did not tell. The actual event had clouded the conscious memory, moving into an unconscious or powerfully negative but subconscious personal belief. When incorrect self-blaming or self-hatred has remained uncovered for many years, the behavioural impact may be observed as a mental illness, unless the onset is finally and consciously exposed. With an opportunity to face the truths about the abuser, therapy can carefully introduce correct and healthy self-beliefs, enabling a proper sense of well-being, the ability to love and accept oneself reclaimed.

The same pain/abuse experienced can elicit quite individually different responses.

You may already appreciate how different personalities are more likely to result in being more vulnerable to negative experiences or inappropriate instructions. It is also evident that the age of the child will also be a key factor. Some children could never respond like the one you may even know, who would simply laugh and confidently want to be even more cheeky!

Back to Tim's response. He was a sensitive, imaginative child, whose love of all things beautiful, strongly surrounded by an innocence so enjoyed about himself and his precious world was suddenly spoilt. His response demonstrated a need to become more and more controlling of his personal world, endeavouring to restore it to some predictable equilibrium. Understanding the strength of his behavioural response to that forgotten trauma became a crucial element in dealing with other compulsive urges that he believed still needed to be controlled.

In addition to knowing more of what might explain the mental health issue, we need to be aware that even when great steps forward are made, such a person may remain vulnerable. An appropriate label may be an appropriate fit for a specific time – it may eventually need to be reassessed, renamed, or even declared to be no longer applicable. Yet an old memory may suddenly erupt when, for example, another disturbing hurdle appears.

Replacing old habits with new ones

Almost a year after his last visit to me, Tim did make another appointment. He reported that everything had been going really well until recently, and he now feared that OCD was going to dominate his life again, and forever – the permanent all-pervasive potential referred to in Chapter 6, contended by Seligman. The issue had grown out of Tim's lack of social confidence. His needing to mix with new associates at a new workplace was a completely new problem, so helping him understand this proved to be an invaluable reassurance. The earlier problem had rested on his childhood responses. These had needed more frequent sessions to affirm new habits, new *adult* beliefs to replace long-standing *childish* beliefs he had to unlearn.

This more recent issue however only warranted two or three sessions to quickly allay his fears, with the path behind no longer needing attention, and his way ahead no longer perceived to be so indelibly distressing. His personality type, as a more intuitive "feeling" idea-driven (idea-ist[5]) person, always sought to *understand* before moving forward. This made him an eager student, though self-doubt was never far away.

But when we think about the differences between Sheryll (mentioned above) and some of the responses made by Michael (mental illness experienced as a result of drug addiction), we continue to ask why that difference exists. Is there, as some research had suggested, an *honesty gene* to be blamed? Or were the parental upbringings in question? Were experiences during crucial developmental stages ones that demanded a response in whatever way they knew how, simply to survive that experience?

Perhaps individual differences as seen in and gauged by a self-report inventory may give us at least a partial answer.

Understand personality

As an aside here, some individual differences identified by trustworthy self-report personality measures may help us see where individuals lie on a broad spectrum of differences, providing a *continuum* between two extremes at either end, but always without the unhelpful negative labels usually resorted to. Using such measures to understand personal and preferred ways of behaving can effectively remove some of the misunderstandings, the self-hate or feelings of blame observed from others' reactions, which often arise through a lack of understanding. We dig deeper into personality in Chapters 12 through 14.

Differences that may suggest mental health issues

There will be times, however, when you are asked to assist a person with a serious mental health issue that makes rational interactions or cognitive approaches quite difficult. Apart from cleverly developed defence mechanisms that block a person's ability to see the truth, there may also be the problem of a *limited capacity* to grasp a more rational explanation. But when you decide to be creative about your "therapeutic" approach of choice, you will discover wonderful alternatives. Like simple rewards for good behaviours: we all know how well even animals can become obedient and faithful friends, based on our quietly consistent behaviours towards what we expect of them, motivated by obvious attitudes of respect and love. Offering positive incentives to change current behaviours will also create more feelings of happiness, either for themselves or for the people who care for them.

How do we work with those said to be mentally unwell?

As mentioned earlier, this question concerning our role as mental health workers remains one that may disturb us. But we are less concerned when clarifying our role if we:

- assess our own abilities with mental ill-health issues
- can make a serious assessment of what can be expected of such a person with particular and inherently consistent behaviours; and
- ensure our assessment capability is counterbalanced by our caring conviction that such a person deserves our respect and care.

Be honest, however: judging such a person as worthy of help, regardless of their behaviour, may still be personally too challenging, especially if the other's personality and attitude seem to radically conflict with our own.

That said, one should never assume that it is impossible to assist change in the unacceptable behaviour of someone exhibiting a mental health issue. But it may take some thinking outside the box for us to offer appropriate relief. Always question whether that particular mental unwellness means there is no hope.

> "Hope is both the earliest and the most indispensable virtue inherent in the state of being alive. If life is to be sustained, hope must remain, even where confidence is wounded, trust impaired."
>
> Erik Erikson[6]

We are not to judge a person's worthiness of help.

We can never be sure how differently individuals may respond to offered support options. Impatience for change in others, however, may suggest a lack of reflection about our own inadequate behaviours! A classic example is recognised in the person found guilty of murder. When a sexual offender against a child joins other prisoners, he is quickly victimised, often regarded as having committed a worse crime than the murderer!

How quickly we can fall into the same pattern, forgetting the principle of "in the same way you judge others you will also be judged"! But when inappropriate behaviour erupts from someone suffering a mental affliction, need for help becomes intensified, and the health professional needs to accept those complexities as part of the task ahead. This is especially the case when engaging other family members in the process, so that maximum support can be encouraged.

The eternal nature–nurture debate

I remember attending one of the very early conferences organised by a group focused on preventing sexual assault and supporting victims. The theme that emerged in most of the sessions clearly demonstrated to me how angry people were, and often indicated a high degree of personal interest associated with getting some revenge. A serious lack of thought was evident about what had led perpetrators to behaving as they did. Some would dismiss the abuser as mentally ill. Others decided that such an abuser most likely had inherited this propensity, and should be treated as worthless and needed to be castrated!

If honest discussion had been conceivable, some individuals might have admitted to there being familial patterns that might lead to a partial excusing of the person on the basis of a genetic disposition. Alternatively, others would have declared that we come into the world with a clean slate, so choices are clearly the individual's responsibility.

In discussing the ever-current nature/nurture question, it was quite disturbing when asked if any present would ever engage in therapy with a perpetrator. To an answer given in the affirmative, most expressed a strong negative reaction. There was little assent to the principle proposed by the compassionate Healer who, when confronting the law-abiding citizens of the day stoning a "sinful" person, said: "the one who is sinless should cast the first stone!"[7]

There seemed to be little cognisance or apparent understanding of most attendees of the sexual assault conference about situations and circumstances that may in various unpredictable ways have hugely impacted on individuals prior to their offending. We must be alert to these potentially crucial elements before we try to help, for these can seriously contribute to why that person sits with us. Compassionate understanding can provide important explanations of at least some of the otherwise unexplainable choices evident in the presenting problematic behaviours.

Skills needed to deal with mental illness

But if we are seriously committed to helping those suffering any issues related to unwellness, whether it has been diagnosed or is just apparent from observations of their dysfunctional or even difficult behaviours, there are some additional skills we need to have.

What would you now list as essential skills? Knowing the plethora of illnesses that we come across in everyday life, be they physical, emotional, mental, or spiritual, we do need to have a greater insight into our own skills, *and* our limitations.

Again, we need to be aware of the impact of both our competencies and personal inclinations. This issue will be considered more deeply in Chapter 18, where we consider the personal needs of those caring for others that often demand more of us than we can give.

REFLECTIVE EXERCISES

- Spend some time thinking about specific people you have difficulty relating to. Is this because of their personalities, their values, or their behaviours? Then think about whether you would find it difficult to work with or even just be caring for them.
- If you knew a diagnosis had been made, such as being depressed, suffering from schizophrenia, or labelled as mentally ill, would that mean you would feel unable to help? Ask yourself what would make you feel that way.
- Could you handle people with a label in the same way as those without such a label? Would seeing that person as just another human being be genuinely likely? In what ways might this not be possible?
- What attitudes might clearly indicate that you were not being professional, let alone showing unconditional love? List your own attitudes, then justify them to someone you respect.
- Ask yourself whether you may need to become more informed about specific illnesses before you realistically can offer to help. Even your own personal *feelings* may stand in the way of assessing whether or not you should help!

- Form your own understanding of what mental health involves. Clarify your understanding of the issues around wellness, well-being, mental health, or mental illness; identify factors that might influence your involvement.

As we've noted that some elements of mental illness have involved addictions, the next chapter will focus on these mental health issues that demand further attention and understanding.

Notes

1 Princess Alice of Battenberg, mother of the late Duke of Edinburgh, was reportedly born congenitally deaf, but whose differentness was later diagnosed as schizophrenia; this saw her committed to a sanatorium for many years. She was a very capable, caring human being, having founded a Greek Orthodox order of compassionate nuns. But her return to a more normal existence became impossible as a result of her years of isolation.

2 You may like to consider Samuel Butler's book *Erehwon* ("nowhere" backwards) from 1872, that satirically suggests that in a Utopia, committed criminals need to be hospitalised, and people with illness be punished by imprisonment!

3 Check out Wikipedia about Milton H Erickson (1901–1980). Here we see it reported that personal struggles clearly increased his valued understanding of the unconscious mind, along with his innovative use of metaphor – all quite inspiring.

4 See https://www.abc.net.au/news/2023-11-18/adhd-diagnosis-ritalin-stimulant-induced-psychosis/103108260.

5 Idea-ist, also used without hyphen, comes from our research on thinking styles; it describes a person who has a rich idea-oriented thinking life with a strong need to understand. See Chapter 13, Ways of Thinking.

6 E H Erikson, *The Erik Erikson Reader*, ed. R Coles (New York: W.W. Norton, 2000). Eric Erikson was a psychoanalytical educational and developmental psychologist. He became renowned for an ego-focused understanding that raised the importance of an individual's identity, and how this can be impacted on by continued societal influences throughout one's life. Hope is seen as inextricably interrelated to identity.

7 John's Gospel 8:7.

Chapter 11

Addictions or habits – good and bad

Addictions are typically assumed to involve some sort of psychological or physiological compulsion to use or to do something. This assumption often brings with it a sense of resignation and helplessness, the solution seen as requiring a diagnosis and therefore complex clinical treatment. In this chapter we encourage readers to understand many addictions as being, at their core, emotionally and/or behaviourally conditioned habits. We explore the empowering that comes when the conceptualisation and management of such addictions as habits has facilitated personal responsibility and control. At the same time, some cases illustrate the effects of chronic physiological dependency on a person's sense of personal identity, with long-term interference on normal developmental experiences: these include parenting styles, problematic attachment, and even abuse. While behavioural training may be part of helping individuals overcome addictions, cognitive considerations such as addressing irrational beliefs are essential to ensure enduring empowerment. Such work, however, is not merely achieved through rational understanding: it needs experiential support such as the use of role-play and Gestalt work.

We would be cognitively and emotionally overloaded if we had to decide every action every day. So we can accept that much of what we do is habitual, though many patterns of our daily living, once established, are not reviewed unless we deliberately set a time to do so. New Year's Eve is one such time, when some plan to start afresh, make new resolutions, determined to develop some good habits and to stop some bad ones. However, maybe you have decided *not* to make New Year resolutions so as not to be faced yet again with an inevitable list of discouraging failures. Habits die hard, they say, and it's so easy to give up!

But it is interesting to note that we don't tend to think of addictions as habits, despite CBT clearly explaining the underlying psychological mechanisms as quintessentially the same. So, are they really the same? We are inclined to

DOI: 10.4324/9781003474746-11

consider habits as things we have some choice and control over, while addictions once formed are those repeated behaviours/actions which largely seem impossible to escape from.

This difference is also seen in our coping. We tend to admit to habits but deny we have an addiction. In life, the more we consider something uncontrollable, the more we are likely to deny it, subconsciously fearing an addiction. Culturally, addiction is seen as a sign of weakness. The term addiction, we suggest, implies a habit, good or bad, to which a person is hopelessly *enslaved*. We also suggest that while addictions present mental health problems, in general there is no necessary explanation in terms of mental illness, though a mental illness may exacerbate or frustrate an addiction in some cases. Again, this illustrates the important point that mental health should not be confused with mental illness.

Accepting personal responsibility for an ingrained bad habit can be challenging, especially where there has been relentless defeat in the past: either rationalisations or excuses have been well formed, or there is secondary gain by maintaining the addiction. These need to be carefully explored and addressed. Let's look at a number of these through the eyes of individuals who confronted their nemesis.

Gambling

Phil had sat down after our pleasant introductions. I was somewhat surprised with the two-word answer I received when I then asked him what brought him in.

"My wife."

"Your wife?"

"Yes, my wife."

"How is it that you are here because of your wife?"

"Bev said I should come and see you."

"And what about you: do *you* think you need to see me?"

"No."

"So, do you at least know what was in your wife's mind in her wanting you to come in to see me?"

"Yes. But I don't agree."

"If you don't think there is any purpose in seeing me, how is it that you have come in anyhow?"

"I do as I am told." His eyes now down and his voice lowered, he sounded serious and embarrassed, rather than mocking or sarcastic in any way.

I reflected. Here was someone who was here because of someone else's agenda. Whatever had driven his wife to suggest that he should come and see me could not be an agenda for us to work on, he having indicated that he rejected that. So, no sense in asking what it was he understood her agenda to be, at least at this stage. His body language however suggested that there was another problem that had driven him to come in. The asking of why at this stage was clearly not useful. Before probing him in that direction, there was a need to build better trust and understanding. I asked him to tell me about himself.

He freely and matter-of-factly told me he was an accountant. He'd lived with his mother until she died five years earlier, on his 55th birthday. Two months later he married Bev, the manager of a small retail outlet. He knew her through his being the tax accountant for the enterprise. It was as if his story was a set of straightforward facts, and though I listened, carefully reflecting along the lines described in Chapters 2–4, I could not get any feedback about how he felt, about *anything*, other than him saying everything was ok. For example, when I probed about how he felt about his mother passing, his answer was again, "Oh that was ok because it was not unexpected: she was old and had cancer, so it was a merciful release."

An interesting observation: while there had been smiles at the pleasant introduction and good and sustained eye contact from him while he shared his story, his incredibly flat affect now suggested that his emotions had been switched off. Was he depressed or perhaps somewhere on a neuro-developmental spectrum? I wanted to know whether Phil expressed feelings about anything, so I left the interpersonal domain and asked him if there were any sports teams he followed. His eyes lit up when he found we barracked for the same team. As we discussed recent games, his emotional expressions were strong, animated, and even full of enthusiasm and excitement. I concluded that in the *interpersonal* domain, he had locked away his feelings.

But I knew a bridge had been built. Crunch time. We needed to confront the elephant in the room: what was it that his wife thought he needed to get professional help with? His demeanour dropped. It was a gamble, but I needed to fit it in before the end of our session. I had judged correctly: enough trust had now been built for him to share.

"She thinks I have a gambling problem. I don't."

In the last ten minutes of the session, the full story came out. He worked hard. Came home mostly around 7 p.m. in time for dinner, and then some TV before bed and an early rise for work. There was not much talk. His wife was an organiser, just like his mum. Outstanding cook. House proud. Every year, mid-winter, Bev went off to Queensland to visit her daughter for a month. This year, however, she had come back to find their joint bank account empty. He explained to her that he had lost it betting, and on the pokies, but was confident he would win it back. When she learned that he could not repay anything from his personal account because that too was now empty, she had become very angry, telling him he had a gambling problem and needed help. But, argued Phil:

"I don't have a gambling problem, just a run of bad luck. I know what I am doing. I will get it back from my earnings, and I know how to win on the horses: I have done it before."

How to engage a person in denial? I also perceived an incredible risk for his clients in regard to any trust accounts he would be managing for them. Somehow a part of him seemed to know he needed help, because there were no protests when I indicated I suspected he had been in this situation before, suggesting he might come in for another session, just to talk that through. Being aware that overcoming addictions requires not only personal ownership of the acknowledged problem, but also social support, I asked if he would be willing to bring his wife along.

Over the ensuing sessions other details became clear: Phil had been the only child of a possessive and controlling single mother. The pattern of playing loose on the pokies as a young adult had started when, each year, he was free from his mother's controls while she was away for a couple of weeks. Phil's wife was horrified to think that she had simply taken over the mother role, control and all!

Addiction such as to gambling can at one level be explained in simple terms of conditioning, so that the treatment needed might be no more than standard straight Cognitive Behaviour Therapy (CBT), as a brief therapy to deal with the here and now. In such, the cognitive work includes teaching about statistical probabilities and likelihoods. For example, many people intuitively believe that a random order of a set of numbers is considered much more likely to win than an ordered or sequential set of numbers like 1, 2, 3, 4, 5, 6.

Interestingly, when put to Phil, he acknowledged that he understood that *either* was just as unlikely. He *knew* that poker machines were actually designed to ensure that the longer one played, the more certain the loss! It became clear that Phil's addictive impulses had been triggered by a sense of there being no external controls, with the result that, lacking *self-control*, his impulsive, previously conditioned behaviour had kicked in. So often this automatic response is the product of controlling, authoritarian parenting (see more on this in Chapter 12) which had kept him the compliant child.

Bringing this to his relatively new relationship needed a form of understanding that challenged the unhealthy roles assumed in their interactions. Consequently, we engaged in couples therapy which involved harnessing Transactional Analysis (TA). Both took to this comfortably. They reviewed, analysed, and learned to interact as adult to adult, rather than as parent to child. Being able to assume an adult role brings with it a sense of responsibility not unlike that which comes instinctively with parenting a newborn baby.

As an aside here, it should be noted that fashions for particular therapeutic systems can exist, and while TA may not be the current fashion, it still can be the most appropriate model providing levers for a situation such as that described here.

In the end, the crisis saw an agenda fulfilled that neither had expected. A couple of years later I came across Phil and his wife walking hand in hand in the local supermarket. To my asking how they were, intending to not solicit anything more than ok, Phil's wife with a grin suggested they should come back to see me. Phil, she said, had become far too inclined to argue, which of course he immediately and strongly protested!

An eating disorder

Moving on to other entrenched behavioural patterns, let us consider how an eating disorder, for example, might benefit from being understood as a bad habit or an addiction. Surely as an eating disorder, anorexia involves deeply embedded problems of identity and self-image. Certainly, these are almost always interwoven as contributing factors, often along with anxiety. But nothing can simply be assumed: there can be quite differing drivers that need to be carefully drawn out, such as guilt and control.

A fifteen-year-old boy diagnosed as suffering from anorexia comes to mind. Note that the word "suffering" has implications in terms of control.

Jeremy was an all-round A+ student who also loved and excelled at athletics and various sports. He was popular at school with both students and teachers. His family were lovingly described as sports "nutters" at their local church where they organised many engaging sporting events. His father, a teacher, coached the local junior football team, and his mother, a dietician originally from India, coached the local adult netball team. Jeremy had a younger brother and sister.

Just after his thirteenth birthday, his mum had noticed Jeremy become more picky about food. She knew that when Jeremy took on something, he could become quite obsessive. A colleague had once asked her if she thought he might have a "somewhat addictive personality". His mother dismissed this at the time, but as his eating habits became more problematic, she had started to wonder.

Being in a health profession can create other problems: from collegial contacts being always available with shared informal advice, to worrying about too many potential explanations!

Soon Jeremy refused to eat any carbs or sugary foods. Was he on a protein kick? Was he getting a buzz out of his dieting? But then his weight, never a problem, started to drop to problematic levels. Mum's attempt to raise the issue with Jeremy met with uncharacteristic sullenness and, if pressed, he told her to mind her own business.

She then spoke to a family therapist at work. As one professional to another, he suggested she might try backing off, since eating disorders often developed from family dynamics and expectations. After all, Jeremy was an eldest child and there could be issues of control for an emerging and competitive teenager. So she pulled right back, working hard to ignore anything to do with eating. It was difficult to educate and encourage both Jeremy's siblings and her husband to stop commenting.

Several months later Jeremy had collapsed while working out at the gym and was taken to hospital. A paediatrician, a GP, a dietician, and a social worker trained in family therapy finally formed a team that also included myself. The question was raised by his mother about whether we thought Jeremy had an addictive personality that could explain his behaviours. A number of other disturbing habits, many previously hidden, had now shown up. These ranged from hours of ball bouncing, sleeping under rather than on his bed, getting up in the middle of the night, and listening to heavy metal music on his Walkman while rolling a ball around his bedroom. Before retiring, he had formed a habit of checking window and door locks around the house. His father asked about the potential explanation of OCD.

Though Jeremy quite happily came along to talk with various team members, he refused to concede that there was any problem. It was his body, his life, and how he ate was his business.

Skiing season was approaching, and Jeremy was clearly looking forward to it. The paediatrician told Jeremy he would not be able to go skiing because of his critical physical condition, which would make him unable to cope with the cold. So before he could possibly go, he would have to weigh in at the hospital over a certain weight.

Jeremy was uncharacteristically really angry when he saw me alone. How dare others control his life! But there was another issue. He was going for confirmation, and his priest had challenged him about not eating enough to sustain his God-given body. He asked me what I thought: was he being sinful? Not for me to answer in any way, I simply turned the question back to him. His answer was straightforward. I did not understand. He just had to do it. While I wanted to ask if he had a reason, instead I asked suggestively, "Has something happened, Jeremy, something traumatic you'd rather not share?" He sat silently for a few moments and then changed the subject to talk about the weekend football match. Intuitively I knew I had touched on something, and his habits and addictions were most likely not a result of OCD but some other personal issue we'd not considered.

Late that evening I received a call from his mother. Jeremy had come home and gone straight to his room, far more withdrawn than usual. As his mother and father were cooking, he had come out, and they expected him as usual to tell them what he would not be eating. But instead, he yelled at them that *they* were obsessed with food. His father gently took hold of him by putting his arm around him, quietly saying they loved him and respected his decisions. He broke away, looked at his mother and burst out crying. Hands now covering his face, amid sobs he asked: "What if you have done something and liked doing it so bad, that even God could never forgive you?"

Over an intense next couple of hours, the story came out. Whenever his parents and siblings had been out, the 18-year-old boy next door had come over and offered Jeremy his favourite chocolate, on condition that Jeremy would have some fun with him. The supposed fun was explicit sexual experimentation, recognised then by his parents as abuse. It had been repeated several times whenever the neighbour noticed Jeremy was home alone.

A number of counselling sessions followed. How did it end? A few years later I was involved in running some study method sessions for year 11 students, and, as is not uncommon, as we walked away from the last session, the organising teacher and I discussed the various students' reactions. We had talked about coping with stress and expectations. To my joy the teacher mentioned Jeremy, reporting him to be one of the most "together" students in the group: focused, capable, determined, and yet easy-going.

We can so easily put bad habits and addictions down to a disorder of one kind or another.

We need to more readily understand a "disorder" as a *descriptive symptom*, not as a trait. Consider for example someone who says, "I am an anorexic" or "I have an addictive personality", "she is a hypochondriac", or "he is such a narcissist". The language suggests that the disorder forms their identity, and as such has trait-like unavoidable causality. As already mentioned in Chapter 10, we need to avoid diagnostic entrapment with consequential disempowerment that engenders a sense of defeat and powerlessness. Over the years we have learned that even when individuals appear stuck, with patience and perseverance, opportunities may arise that bring an enduring or a one-off traumatic event to the surface, needing to be removed like a festering splinter.

Traits and habits: self-management

Consider Tamara, a young mum of two under-fives, who had been battling anorexia and at times bulimia for the last ten years, apparently since she was 14. Years of unsuccessful counselling and therapy had, she said, confirmed to her that her anorexia was part of her genetic makeup, or at least a predisposition that would be triggered by any stress. To exonerate herself from any guilt, she had simply told herself, "I am an anorexic, and I cannot help that. I just need to manage it."

From her history it was clear that she had worked through many irrational beliefs, so could gain reasonable control using a number of behavioural management techniques. Her understanding was that she had been born with a propensity to anorexia. The initial onset, she said, had been triggered by stress, "discovered" with her previous counsellor. This initial stress had been experienced when, as the eldest child of four, she had increasingly felt responsible for holding her family together. Her mother suffered frequent psychotic episodes that necessitated hospitalisation. Her father had withdrawn, working ever longer hours, leaving her in charge.

Now that Tamara was again experiencing a particularly difficult struggle with eating issues, the CBT techniques that otherwise gave her control were not working. She was determined to gain control. We reviewed the techniques she had been taught, then explored any irrational beliefs. I was impressed by her honesty and openness, not least in her determination to identify any potential secondary gain. Ever in control, she asked whether relaxation might help. She had tried various forms, but had always found that she could not relax. Trying to relax was inevitably interrupted by a loud stream of conscious thoughts, including an urgent sense of needing to *not* let go, needing to remain in control.

Relaxation through tensing

Identifying issues of control that are central to so many suffering with anorexia, I suggested to Tamara that we could try a session of relaxation using a technique where she would stay completely in control. An explanation needed me to demonstrate how this worked: I asked her to take out her smartphone, and, without turning it on, to close her eyes and imagine it to be a remote control.

"Simply squeeze the sides firmly to turn off whatever we are doing – I will be watching your hand closely. You are in complete control. Tapping the screen with your other hand once means keep going and twice means pause. Let's practise."

After practising, I asked her if she felt in control. She responded, smilingly, that most certainly and surprisingly, even with her eyes closed, she did! While she held her inactive phone, "directing" the speed through pauses, we were able to move through a conventional relaxation session. Purposefully this did not start with asking her simply to relax, but rather by really tensing up a part of her body (starting at the scalp and forehead and moving progressively down) and then, when everything was held in what was almost insufferable tension, to let everything go, focusing again through the various parts of her body.

The taps on the phone worked well. I could see that she went into a comfortable relaxed state. Whenever she tapped the screen once, I would quietly encourage her to enjoy "controlling herself, leading into an ever-deeper relaxation" and to allow her imagination to bring up pictures that she found relaxing. About seven minutes in, she suddenly tapped twice vigorously, then again twice, and then squeezed the sides. I had meant to guide her back to reality gently, but here she had brought herself back in a hurry, looking as if in shock – not what I had hoped for.

Powerful insights gained through guided imagery

It was clear that Tamara was a person for whom strong cognitive control was the way she usually managed to be in charge. I asked her if she would like to share what she had experienced, ever aware that she needed to *feel* in control.

"When you got me to walk along that beach, well, that woman, walking the other way, that was my mother! She looked so well, didn't she! But then, did you see, she ignored me, she walked right past as if she didn't want or *couldn't* even recognise me!"

In the debriefing, as Tamara moved further back to the present reality, she came to realise that I had neither suggested the content nor been present on the beach! The session however gave us both a clear understanding of how her mother's mental health issues had impacted on her.

She now grasped her own capabilities and, when needed, was able to take herself off into an imaginary world by using Gestalt techniques, or to revisit the past where she could imagine talking to her mother. Particularly powerful were the sessions where she was also able to imagine talking to herself as a child, comforting the child within[1] and dispelling any unconscious irrational beliefs, such as being unlovable.

Gestalt techniques

These techniques allow a person to retain a strong sense of control and increased empowerment. There was now no need to challenge Tamara's strongly defended belief of anorexia as a trait she'd been born with. In effect, symptom abatement did its own work. Some twelve months later Tamara returned and reported having developed a routine of relaxation and self-talk to which she attributed her success:

no more problems with eating. She clearly felt control with a sense of ownership. Smilingly, at the close of her session, she said she would be back for another set of techniques when these lost their effectiveness. I gently suggested she might like to think in terms of "if" rather than "when". She had removed the splinter of irrational beliefs associated with a failed attachment to her mother. The newly acquired skill of healthy self-talk can be an effective part of coping with other everyday life stressors.

Tamara's case not only illustrates the problem of considering disorders as trait-like, but also points to techniques that effectively allow the use of imagination to reach deep and non-cognitively into the subconscious. Much counselling can benefit from going beyond the rational, didactic, and behavioural. Visualisation, imagination, and talking to the inner child/person can all break through with relief, whereas rationality alone may simply confront well-built, indestructible defence mechanisms.[2]

Hoarding and denial

Let us consider an example of this common habit, and its denial. Robert arrived in a distressed state. His wife of 50 years had announced she was leaving him. Yes, he was 75! He had worked all his life, he said, and still worked to ensure they were secure. It soon became clear that, to that day, Robert had gone to his small factory seven days a week, sometimes from seven in the morning until seven at night. How could his wife walk out when this work was, he said, all for her, the children, and grandchildren? He had been talked into getting help by his eldest son, seeing his parents totally incapable of resolving anything, but who himself had been helped by psychological insights. Robert came in first, to clearly put *his* point of view!

Couples work was called for. Experience has taught us so many times that there may be three stories around any partnership: two individual and at times irreconcilable narratives, and a third shared narrative when the couple is asked to present together.

Maude was clear and direct. Robert had never been there for her, their children, or their grandchildren. The garden was now too large, the house rambling, so she wanted to move to a small unit. Robert however had a large shed and garage on the property filled with "gunna-do" projects that she said were all about him. Robert started going through the projects he had been planning in order to make life easier for Maude. Maude responded that *she* was just *his* excuse for hoarding. It became clear that most of Robert's time was spent sorting and organising his hoarding. His factory was so filled with "stuff" that he also maintained three lock-ups in a local storage centre.

Any challenges to his hoarding addiction met with his justification in terms of some worthwhile intended project, creative ideas running wild. It was soon apparent that he rarely got beyond either managing his hoard or acquiring some new piece for his collection. There was simply no time to carry out any projects other than a trickle of jobs that still came into his factory.

The hoarding addiction had clearly become an end in itself, justified by its potential purpose in terms of projects.

Question: How would you break through so that Robert would be able to recognise an addiction and be willing to deal with it? Maude had finally given up, with her own needs and frail health meaning that she could no longer cope in their shared world.

Motivation and reality

The old motivation pops up again: but the look on Robert's face when I asked him what he expected to be doing in five and then ten years' time said it all. There was a stunned silence. Clearly the reality of the future was not to be considered, and was firmly blocked. Any contemplation of it was defensively denied. It threatened his hoarding addiction.

We didn't talk in terms of addiction, however. Noting that he already needed a walking stick, after saying that nothing needed to change, I asked him if he knew any 80- to 95-year-olds, and what they were able to do day to day. Maude offered the names of three of their old friends, all in nursing homes. It was too hard to contemplate. Robert stood up, grabbed his walking stick, and walked out of the session without a word.

Sadly, Robert was diagnosed a few weeks later with a particularly aggressive form of cancer from which he died within a few months. Maude, grief-stricken, came in for a number of sessions, needing to debrief about their final days together. Apparently, after walking out of his last session, Robert had said nothing to Maude, but to her surprise had started to clean up his garage and shed at home.

You can see how addiction over time can become well defended, at least at the conscious level. Reality testing is an essential step before acknowledging an addiction. Realising and accepting the destructive effects of an addiction is also needed to drive a sufficiently powerful motivation for the person to consciously accept problem ownership and then to take responsibility to make changes.

Addiction – a complex interaction of the psychological and the physiological

Addiction, however, is seldom simply psychological. We need to reflect again on the examples of problems associated with alcohol already mentioned, such as that of Colin (Chapter 7, under Reactive Depression). There we saw alcohol used as a soft drug, as self-medication for depression and PTSD. Over time an inevitable physiological dependence develops, even though more slowly than chasing the dragon that can be set off after just one dose of hard drugs, like heroin. The *psychological* can be explained by conditioning: immediate rewards experienced and remembered, supported by irrational beliefs or rationalising. The *physiological* addiction however can be compared to a physical thirst, clamouring to be satisfied.

Seemingly innocuous activities can become physiologically driven addictions. Running through the pain barrier can release endorphins. Comfort food, computer games, pornography, and nicotine are just some of the substances and activities that can provide a short-term escape, with regrets often following. Psychological factors alone, even with understanding and willpower, are not enough to deal with such dependencies, though commitment and willingness to take ownership and responsibility are essentials for positive outcomes. In all of these, any attempt to gain control over a problematic addiction also needs to take into account the physiological factors.

A brief comment needs to be made here: we see the individual as always a part of a wider community, so that personal needs in relation to addictions always demand our consideration of how such addictions impact on connected others.

As in most cases, including those mentioned earlier, like Michael (Chapter 10), we recognise how addictions have such destructive effects on more than the individual involved – a societal impact that is still largely growing rather than receding.

REFLECTIVE EXERCISES

- Summarise from the cases just considered: if we name any one thing that people do – *that* can become an obsession or an addiction that is problematic.
- When doing something starts to control us, we lose a sense of choice, and we have a problem. The *drivers* for bad habits and addictions are inevitably some sort of a cocktail of physical biochemical addictions and social factors.

In the cases we have reviewed here, and in many examples given in earlier chapters, consider the following statements, and how you might be ready and able to personally apply these:

- Addressing issues of control and empowerment for taking responsibility can be seen as crucial. Doing so with *more than* straight rationalistic cognitive/behavioural approaches is often the only way forward.
- Alternatives, like using imagination to reach into the subconscious, can impel clients to dance around any well-entrenched defence mechanisms to find unexpected solutions.
- Good outcomes are not just due to personal inner work or countering behavioural conditioning. There are clear indications that suggest a need to incorporate crucial *social factors* will also provide support for change.
- Understand why having and building good relationships is so important, not only for dealing with addictions and undesired habits, but for instituting alternative good habits that impact physical and mental health.

More in Chapter 14 about this. But for now, the next chapter considers more fully what knowing and accepting ourselves, and all that identity implies, *before* moving into how that self-knowledge may impact our relationships.

Notes

1 Gestalt Technique associated with relieving effects of childhood trauma are described in J Roodenburg and E Roodenburg's novel, *Psychological Digs in Paradise* (Mona Vale, Sydney: Ark House Press, 2022).

2 Look up reputable sources on defence mechanisms on the internet, such as on healthline.com or PsychologyToday.

Chapter 12

Personality and relationships

Throughout this book, numerous allusions have been made to how personality plays a part in the behaviour or mental health issue being discussed. This chapter further explores the understanding of individual differences, with important questions that require answers about what is commonly understood as personality. It also looks at what research has been able to identify: both the uniqueness experienced as well as the factors that are held in common by other unique individuals. Additional elements like values collisions that aggravate potential breakdowns in relationships are explored. Similarly, significant personality differences, particularly when seen as extreme scores on a continuum, will have more of an effect on how well we navigate relationship issues, and on individual choices made for career paths. Using our preferred way of thinking and behaving does not however mean that we cannot use the non-preferred side, just as we can learn to use our left hand if the right hand suffers an injury. Learning styles can also be reflected in our personal choices; but being open to learning will grow our adaptability to cope in various situations, and needs to be encouraged, not shunned.

Personality: traits and dispositions

When we reflect on personality, we often refer to distinctive patterns of behavioural and emotional expressions that seem to cluster in a unique way in any one person, forming a personality we either love to be with or not! Personality Psychology[1] has long recognised such patterns as dispositions,[2] with consistent traits, to varying degrees, observed to be relatively stable over time within individuals, particularly in certain contexts or predictable situations. Dispositions are thought to reflect many underlying traits, for example introversion or conscientiousness, and may each involve a range of differential abilities; they are also often considered to be interwoven in various combinations of cognitive ways of thinking.

Mapping these factors scientifically has been the work of dispositional psychology, which over years has harnessed sophisticated statistical and more

DOI: 10.4324/9781003474746-12

recent qualitative analyses to ensure construct validity.[3] In short, to be valid, each of the constructs needs to be unique, that is, distinct from one another, yet together as a set of measures, these descriptives need to capture a full and comprehensive range of differences.

Results from developing personality indicators, questionnaires and ability tests using psychometrics have converged with research in neuroscience. Well-established psychometric instruments based on the Big Five personality and the CHC ability models[4] are now used with confidence in both personal and workplace situations.

Chapter 13 will also give you an additional more recently developed self-report questionnaire that you might find helpful to differentiate particular traits, specifically to better understand your own typical way of thinking (WOT). But first, let's ask: how does understanding personality really impact building and maintaining good relationships?

Individuals need to connect

Today we are surrounded by people crying out for connections, as an understandable human response to feeling alone. It becomes particularly needful in those who have experienced limited opportunities for forming good trustworthy relationships. Sometimes this cry has grown out of disrupted home lives, often caused by people having had to relocate, whether for work or other more personal reasons. Whether through ill health or curfews imposed such as during COVID, extended time alone can block important opportunities to relate closely. There is now global recognition of an increased sense of isolation for many people, regardless of age.

Some disruptions are created by serious circumstances, with the result that where abuse has occurred or families are separated, reconciliation of their differences seems impossible. Acrimonious resolutions are frequently made that impact those directly involved; this can also mean that children, through no fault of their own, are left to pick up what pieces they can, trying to make sense of the break-up. Strong repercussions from broken relationships are often experienced by the extended family members, like grandparents. Even good close relationships are often severed by a physical distance occasioned by war, natural disasters, and subsequent migration, with many finding it increasingly difficult to maintain good relations.

Relationship breakdowns

As more relationships today fall by the wayside, we are left asking: how much time do people spend in reflecting on what went wrong? Seemingly, many don't ever seriously get to the *why* and *how* questions! Often this is explained by the fact that emotions are so high that the *rational* answers required cannot even become obvious. Various excuses are given, and of course include the insistence that it is always someone else's fault!

> *Brief reflection: what is top of your list of strong reasons as to why so many relationships are not able to last?*

Having read the foregoing cases, you will have observed that the many issues are complex, with a variety of factors contributing to common well-being issues that demand attention. I'm sure that you will have registered many examples throughout this book where communication styles often become the basis for unhappy relationships, as seen in Chapter 4, for example: I- versus You-messages. You will also have noted one other consistent problem: a serious lack of understanding of the differences observed and experienced by individuals and between people, despite good intentions to just get on with each other.

Let's imagine someone whose relationships always make you feel uncomfortable. Let's call her Thea, a strong-looking woman though she identifies herself as not very confident, and she usually backs down in an argument. Now imagine her partner of many years – a small guy who presents as someone who wouldn't hurt a mouse. Yet in getting to know Ed more, you find out that he is often very aggressive, frequently puts Thea down, always correcting her statements, resulting in dissenting interactions that inevitably she withdraws from!

What is your initial reaction to this couple's way of relating? Embarrassment? Dislike of the aggressor? Pity for Thea? Do you perhaps want to correct or even chasten Ed? Decide it's a relationship doomed? You may even wonder how the relationship has survived so long.

Poor relationships can survive

As you leave Thea and Ed's way of relating, let the idea emerge that maybe, just maybe, their decision to stay in that relationship suits both; how *you* see it and feel about it is irrelevant. Not only have they perhaps become habituated to the way it works, but in fact the different personal weaknesses or feelings of inadequacy are compensated for by how the other seems so strong. For some, it seems so much easier to put up with what is, rather than risk making changes – remember Cheryl and Graham (Chapter 5) and for different reasons, Marlene and Jeff (Chapter 9).

If we reflect on the many relationships we engage with, let's again think about our own personal preferences for a moment. For instance, how well do *you* appreciate spending time with friends who are quite different from you? Have you perhaps instinctively understood the title of the book *Opposites Attack*,[5] noting that "attract" is crossed through, and replaced with "attack"? And yet, as mentioned in Chapter 14 on identity, people today seem to prefer to connect in groups, in tribes, feeling comfortable listening to or expressing views with similarly thinking and acting people, and who then act accordingly, particularly when engaging through social media. With the rise of search engines, an associated phenomenon has been identified as confirmation bias,[6] where agreement with the tribe simply confirms beliefs.

As with Thea and Ed, strong differences between people can make relationships challenging. However, such opportunities can be incredibly enriching, if embraced and appreciated, and when the sharing between differently oriented people occurs without fear of being criticised, threatened, or made to feel inadequate. Before such openness between people can really blossom, however, there needs to be an honest understanding about those differences, and how these can best be handled.

Lack of understanding of individual differences

Any lack of understanding of personal differences can cause people to retreat into their safe bias-sharing enclosures or silos. Unfortunately, this can also create another potential problem, one of imbalance: seeing the world through a singular one-eyed perspective.

> *Close one eye for a second, and then close the other: notice how much is missed by using only one eye!*

Having similar personalities (see Chapter 13 with Jamie and Melissa) does not guarantee that everything runs well. But an *inability* or *unwillingness* to see things through another's distinct perspective can be the basis of so many arguments, and inevitable bitter disagreements. Historically this is universally documented on all sides of politics, and in frequent wars that continue to destroy our world: one group trying to powerfully dominate another, in complete contradiction of their expressed need for peaceful coexistence.

All this happens in spite of widespread educational opportunities, and with knowledge today just a Google away! Knowledge indeed benefits us when intertwined with wisdom, understanding, respect, and an appreciation of the very differences that make us unique beings. But as indicated by the variety of tools used with individual issues, we affirm our commitment to the very praxis that must at all times be undergirded by our phronesis. The will *to understand* must be effectively underscored by the necessary value of treating others as we would like to be treated. This highlights the importance of acceptance, with certain positive values of mutual respect, which, when combined with appropriate modelling, often encourages others to behave in like manner.

Of course, there are many other reasons that frequently contribute to breakdowns in relationships. I'm reminded of Dawn and Roberta, two women who'd been friends as teenagers but met again some thirty years later. Both were lonely after relationship failures, and since both were experiencing a midlife crisis, they had thrown in their city jobs, wanting to achieve the perfect, peaceful, pleasant more rural life together.

Values collision

They discovered, however, that they had very different values. Dawn was a saver, meaning that hard-earned money was to be carefully used only when really needed. Roberta on the other hand loved spending! She loved going out and going on holidays, whereas Dawn loved the quiet of home, tending her chickens while caring for their garden. Such a clash of values may be resolved with commitment and love, openness to negotiation, and modifying one's strongly held beliefs in considered awareness of what is being sacrificed. But for these women, having already spent many years each living very different lifestyles, the cost was too great. They were unwilling to give up their personal values in favour of the *other's* expectations for a future "good life" together. Understanding their personality differences in itself did not compensate for their clash in values, finally deemed insurmountable.

We all have ready examples that demonstrate what happens when love wonderfully covers over relationship dilemmas. But deep problem areas between people are often ignored, excused, or treated as invisible, particularly where denial explains the issue away – until it is impossible to pretend that things are getting better. At such points of disagreement, many an individual decides they only have two options: search for someone to sort out the other's problem, or to walk away, cutting their losses. We've cited examples of these in earlier chapters.

If you have not experienced this dilemma yourself, you may have come across it between other people you know. And when a conflict is experienced between three mutual friends, of which you are one, another problem arises. Depending on where the conflict lies, you may have to choose which person remains your friend. Or if your role is to be the outsider, there's a strong imperative to remain impartial, so that other skills become essential. Let's look again at examples of people in such circumstances who came to see me, some with clear agendas of separation, while others genuinely wanted to know what best to do.

Individual differences need acknowledgement

We've already mentioned Sam, way back in Chapter 2, who struggled with knowing who he was and where he was heading. Remember his intention to walk away from his wife, although he felt quite uncomfortable about that option. Clarity regarding the real issues enabled some new workarounds that early on helped him to stay in the relationship; the next steps allowed him to work at rebuilding their relationship. Sometimes this suggests a valuable ganging up against a problem together which can be so helpful. What else made that change possible? Well, in addition to the exposure of long-held beliefs that propped up some bad habits, Sam was really committed to unearthing the truth, which was married to a healthy determination to implement his new understanding. For Sam, this became possible when he recognised and accepted their individual differences. When his new perceptions were honestly shared with his wife without fear, together they could face the necessary changes.

Misunderstandings related to individual differences

You will meet young Joey again in Chapter 13. A boy who rarely spoke unless spoken to, yet Joey clearly had a wonderful range of words whenever he did speak. His mother Sondra reported that he had quickly learned to read even before commencing school, but clearly he disliked the sociability expected of him in class.

There are several points about that relationship that are relevant here. For example, whenever Sondra had spoken about Joey, it was as if she did not really know her son. She just knew that he was very different from her, which bothered and frustrated her immensely. I had observed that Joey was obviously verbally quite able, and as a nine-year-old he had been able to read and answer the WOT Child version for himself. The successful ongoing counselling allowed me to make further important observations through discussing the results of the questionnaire. It was apparent that Sondra's son was not suffering from a mental disability, but rather from *her* lack of understanding. She had eventually admitted that Joey's father had also been a mystery to her, and with his leaving the family three years before, she had never considered how his personality profile might have been similar to her son's.

Compared with that of Tom (Chapter 1), as another boy who ran away from home, Joey's initial *need* for psychological assistance had a very different causal basis, his being specifically about increased need for time to think alone. But it is important to note that the outcomes were similarly and powerfully related to the parent's lack of understanding of individual differences. Joey could become less isolated by his mother's greater understanding of him. In turn, by understanding her own very different personality, Sondra then greatly benefited from understanding her part in what had contributed to the breakdown of her adult partnership.

Personality differences

> *Individual differences are individual dispositions that may best be conceived of as personality preferences.*

So, let's think further about individual differences that may best be conceived of as personality preferences. For example, I like being flexible, adaptable – but you may prefer to be organised, to make plans, and determinedly need to sit with decisions made. Or, you may say you are very sociable, and naturally quite extroverted, hating to have to spend too much time alone. Yet when you think about it, your sibling, born of the same parents, with the same upbringing, seems very *un*comfortable about having to share with a group of known people, let alone be asked to speak with strangers! Likewise, if we think about our learning styles: do you perhaps prefer listening to YouTube videos or podcasts, with clear instructions about how and what to do? Or, as the fact you are reading this book suggests, perhaps you value time to think at your own speed, allowing time for loads of questions that explore the *meaning* behind what is written?

One young man comes to mind, a university student who was keen but struggling to keep up with assignments. Craig loved learning but mostly interactively. He was also so busy interacting socially that he frequently left all written work too late to complete on time. When a personality inventory had him explore his preferred way of learning, he quickly understood his problem. As someone who was a strong extrovert, which explained his social needs, he also became aware of his inclination to be spontaneous, rather than take the more planned approach needed. Yes, this simple self-awareness created a choice for Craig to accept as his responsibility: to *plan* essential things, while also leaving time and space for the spontaneity that was so important for him!

I'd like to suggest that understanding our individual personalities can form a basis on which we can predict *in general* how we are *likely* and *prefer* to respond to the circumstances we face in life, though of course exceptions will occur. The predilection or preference for how we think or act does not put us in a box, controlling us, but rather allows for a more automatic response, unless we need to think about an alternative. For example, as Sheryll (in Chapter 10) gradually came to better understand and accept herself, she could more wittingly make decisions for herself, rather than depend on others to either defend, protect, or alternatively take control of her, as her old practice had been.

Knowing ourselves means we can be prepared for, and less likely to be shocked by, our automatic responses. Understanding *others'* personalities can also make a huge contribution to how effectively they may be encouraged to cope with life's demands. Completing an inventory that highlights individual *strengths* can be so affirming, especially when it alerts a person to counteract the weaker traits that have often been uppermost in their self-perceptions.

Personality impacts on mental health

> *Many mental health issues may well be better handled if understood as individual differences.*

Understanding individual differences may better explain "oddities" in people, particularly if such people are on the outer extremes of a range of what personality measures claim to measure, rather than considering such extremes as a form of mental illness. For example, some surveys or indicators of personality may suggest how extroverted or introverted you are, or how feeling/non-feeling you prefer to be. Other indicators refer to how imaginative/creative an "ideas" person you are, where, at the other extreme of that spectrum, for the "realist" the truth is always considered to be fact, black or white, never grey. All measures of personality try to encapsulate the essence of what is distinctive about an individual.

May I share with you another example of this? A capable intelligent lady in her late thirties, Annika initially had sought help over several serious family issues that had greatly worried her, causing her depression and many anxieties. Several months had elapsed since she reported that she had happily resolved these issues: she had become well practised at relaxation exercises, often confidently doing these to maintain a healthy equilibrium in her busy life as a working mum.

In this later appointment, however, Annika revealed an embarrassing habit of totally misspelling words that even her nine-year-old could spell – and the worst part was that she didn't even notice when she made these mistakes, until pointed out by others. When the current relaxation session included thinking about writing, she became very focused on a time in her life during her teenage years. Quietly reflective, she reported what it was like when her parents had moved, when at aged 14, Annika had been sent to the local Technical Secondary school. Having migrated from the Middle East a few years earlier, and with a limited English language facility, her parents had wanted their daughter to quickly gain skills so that she could start to earn good money for the family. They showed little understanding of how intellectually bright Annika was, with no real knowledge of attitudes that often prevailed among other adolescents deemed only clever enough to require a basic, practical education.

As a consequence, Annika reported how she had often felt very left out. Her questioning of her teachers demonstrated her own academic thinking abilities; this led to classmates making fun of her, believing she was "sucking up" to teachers. This earned her no friends, though her teachers thought well of her.

But you may ask, how does personality relate to this issue for Annika? Well, firstly, if she had been less concerned about others – more introverted and thus less dependent on social acceptance – Annika would have been less likely to have reacted to criticism/non-acceptance by peers. Secondly, during my earlier sessions, when her own mental health was suffering badly, her suicidal ideations had been successfully confronted *largely* due to understanding her personal preferences and ways of thinking. Her strong imaginative abilities had often overwhelmed any awareness of reality, confusing her to a point of distrust of self and others. During those earlier in-depth sessions, exploration of her personality had enabled *personal* acceptance of her Real Self, with appreciation of her strengths then outweighing the previous negative attitudes that had been quite depressing.

Now as an adult, focused on her odd spelling problem, Annika relaxed into reflecting back quite deeply on her school experiences. She remembered a point in time when she had actually *decided* she needed to seem "dumb" if her classmates were to accept her. She remembered she had then started deliberately spelling words incorrectly. She remembered often being laughed at, but after a time, their attitudes had changed, and with her new friends no longer feeling threatened by her, they had begun treating her as one of them.

Oddness reframed as positive attributes

By looking again at her personal preferences, using the Ways of Thinking inventory, Annika recognised her need was to *understand*, rather than just be given the facts. This session became a powerful new high point of self-acceptance. Alerted to a part of herself that had creatively solved her aloneness problem as a teenager, she now engaged that same part to change her habitual "can't spell" behaviour to one that matched her being an intelligent adult. Confronted by new enlightened understanding, that responsible part of Annika now made a significant change. She was determined to change the unconscious *childish* commitment to appearing illiterate, to an acceptance of her exciting new *mature adult* understanding that her abilities be celebrated; this meant that she no longer suffered from internally conflicting feelings.[7] Questions and self-doubts that she had needed to explore but not known how were now grasped with great relief.

At a future session, Annika revealed that her spelling was incredibly no longer an embarrassment to her – and no longer an embarrassment to her clever children! This is an extraordinary but true story that again demonstrates the power of thinking, even to generate habitual behaviours that are not even consciously understood. At times such internal self-talk does need to be consciously acknowledged, but when accepted and acted upon, it can generate powerful and positive associated behaviours.

Individual differences

> *Knowing and accepting how we all differ can generate much in terms of relating well with others.*

I hope you will look back over the characters from preceding chapters whose cases highlight the benefits in gaining insights not just about how we all differ, but even more in how we might deal with people who may be quite challenging.

It is also important to note that personality traits or preferences will provide some of our understanding, even about how differently individuals cope with life. But as already mentioned in a number of the clients considered, their *abilities* also needed to be explored, so that, with appropriate guidance, clarity about their own goals and aspirations could also be appreciated. We will turn to these later, and particularly in the Chapter 15.

However, values, beliefs, and behaviours deemed acceptable or otherwise cannot explain all that we need to consider when there is conflict. Psychology, particularly within the framework of individual differences, has long enjoyed looking at what evidence there is for understanding characteristic traits and aptitudes in people. It has also been committed to a greater understanding of *generalities* that may explain how predictably some individuals behave, yet often quite differently from others who *also* exhibit their own regularly predictable behavioural patterns – each reliable within certain contexts and situations.

Concluding this chapter

It is beyond the scope of this book to wander into the broader historic and current mix of psychological foci that have formed theories about how and why certain behaviours can best be understood. Some of these home in on hereditary elements; some have preferred to think about environmental impacts on individuals and their behavioural choices. However, even from the evidence we have given of the broad continuum of individual differences that demand our understanding, it is possible to identify certain patterns of behaving. These can both help us understand past behaviours of an individual and may also provide some predictability about that individual's future behaving.

While we each have varying strengths across our different dispositional traits, we also have traits in common with many others. Take for example the well-known traits of extroversion versus introversion, or Idea-ism versus Realism (see Chapters 13 and 14), which run from one pole to its opposite. We each can readily recognise that we fluctuate somewhere within a small range on the continuum, often adapting to situations and circumstances.

It is hoped that the reader now understands our assumptions: personality is not like the old "mask" idea of a persona that is put on, to cover the real person, but rather describes an individual's psychological and enduring qualities that best distinguish that person from another whose personality is similar in some respects, but quite different in others. There are many and varied forms of assessment that give important definitive descriptors that are so helpful to understand about individuals. Do seek these out, for yourself if not for others.

When personality-related behaviours are not understood, however, they can mistakenly be interpreted as suggesting that a person is "being obstreperous", or simply "trying to be difficult". Indeed, some may be labelled as mentally deficient. Such differences do demand close and deferential attention, rather than the expectation that such an individual *should* think/act like "normal people" or, even worse, "like I do"! But even when respect is apparent, there will still be other factors that contribute to ineffective or unhappy relations.

REFLECTIVE EXERCISES

Many relational issues can simply be around miscommunications, and these inevitably need to be teased out.

Reflect on some that you have experienced. Are they directly associated with:

- Personality preferences?
- patterns of speech gained from within their family?
- Values/beliefs collisions?

If you have not done so before now, perhaps it's time to consider what other factors you may have observed in struggling relationships, that readily become mixed up with personality characteristics. Even differences in natural abilities can be misunderstood, and so can create resentful barriers that spoil relationships! We hope the later chapter on learning difficulties, Chapter 15, may shed more light on this issue.

Notes

1 Consider any textbook on personality, such as D Cervone and L A Pervin, *Personality: Theory and Research* (Hoboken, NJ: Wiley, 2018). Also worth exploring are a number of online Big Five personality tests with good feedback.
2 Look up "dispositional psychology" for more details.
3 See K Slaney, *Validating Psychological Constructs: Historical, Philosophical, and Practical Dimensions* (London: Palgrave MacMillan, 2017).
4 Details of these are readily available via an internet search; we recommend Wikipedia.
5 J Mayhall and C Mayhall (1992) *Opposites Attack* (Colorado Springs: Navpress, 1992).
6 Confirmation bias abounds; conspiracy theories abound, confirmed from the tribes' "evidence".
7 St Paul's well-known passage on love read in many weddings is a great reflection: childish ways needing to be replaced by adult ways: see 1 Corinthians 13:11.

Chaper 13

Ways of thinking

Research has provided interesting insights into individual differences that are linked to our inherent ways of thinking. These are distinct from, yet clearly interwoven with, our personality and abilities. Idea-ists are reflective of those who value understanding beyond a focus on practical details, with creative ideas often reaching outside the box! On the other hand, Realists find details most important, wanting to make sure these are correct; their thinking is clearly based on what can be seen, touched, or handled. The differences become even more complex if such ways of thinking involve a characteristic of being aware of and accepting the importance of emotions. Ways of Thinking (WOT) will also be expressed differently when individuals are either more strongly introverted or extroverted. Examples also provide evidence of the broader issues of decision making that impact differently on Idea-ists than on Realists. One solution to effectively deal with this difficulty is discussed, utilising a decision-making list of the pros and cons to clarify a way forward.

Have you noticed how quickly we make decisions about who we *like*, based on how they typically behave? If you reflect on the person who is now your best friend, did you always think about him or her so positively? Surely, as a relationship develops, we become more aware of something we call differences, not just in what we typically like doing, but in the way we think. This is not always obvious, so taking time to dig in more deeply makes it easier to say what we can predict about how others may think about certain things. Some of this will relate to how well an individual acts in accordance with their own understanding of who they really are, and how confidently they can express their views. This will also be affected by whether their self-acceptance allows their *Real* Self not to contradict or be in continual conflict with their *Ideal* or *Expected* Self (see Chapter 14 for more on this).

In knowing who we are, it is helpful to have a means of understanding how we are like some people and different from others: in personality, in abilities,

DOI: 10.4324/9781003474746-13

or in our personal ways of thinking about things. Such understanding has an impact on not only what we think of ourselves, but also our likes and dislikes in relationships, and of course then also influences the way we build relationships.

Differences in ways of thinking: Idea-ist versus Realist

Lack of such understanding can be illustrated in the case of a young boy, Joey, mentioned last chapter, who at age nine would no longer speak, at least to anyone in his family or at school. Joey would climb in under his bed at home and read. When it came to homework, he would happily write answers, but he had suddenly refused to speak. In lieu of speech, he would only nod a "yes" or a "no" to those questions he chose to answer (such as would he like some dinner?), but simply went blank when asked anything personal. His mother Sondra thought that she had heard him talking to himself when the door to his bedroom was closed. With homework an indicator, however, we discovered that Joey also had no difficulty filling in questionnaires, so this became a way of engaging him, along with playing pencil and paper games like noughts and crosses and hangman.

> *There is a similarity here to another young boy, Tom, from Chapter 1, but whose silence was due to emotional issues not being understood or addressed . . . refresh your memory!*

But in Joey's case, were there really some indicators of mental illness, you may ask? Maybe selective mutism, or as a response to some abuse? There certainly appeared to be issues of control. One of the questionnaires he completed was the Ways of Thinking (WOT) Inventory (see later) which showed some extreme scores that warranted an alert of a potential health issue. For example, his very *low* preference scores on *reality* checks was in obvious contrast to *strong* scores on what he preferred to imagine. His strong scores for *internal* thinking suggested a need for private space, indicating that social contacts were most likely quite stressful for him. Such factors were a surprise to his single mother yet so important to grasp, as she was the person most entrusted with helping Joey develop a *balanced* potential for another way of looking at and experiencing life. In contrast to her son, Sondra was an exceptionally extroverted professional lady, who expressed most of her thinking out loud, with little inclination to do other than accept the facts as given. In addition, unlike her more "idea-ist" son, she was also a strong "realist" needing to *do* something for her son, while Joey simply needed to understand!

Importance of knowing personality preferences

As an aside, it is important to say again that completing a personality type assessment tool such as the WOT or a Big Five personality assessment does *not* box a person, but rather helps create a picture that identifies a person's preferred way of thinking and operating. An understanding of how we are similar or different can also be a tremendous help to people who are mystified about differences in social interactions.

In this case, Sondra had such an outgoing personality with a strong social need to express her factual thoughts aloud that she had not considered her preferred need to talk as being completely opposite to her son. As a deeply internal thinker who cogitated on many ideas which, at the age of nine, were becoming more and more abstract, Joey needed increased time to think internally. With only him and his loquacious mother at home, he had simply become overloaded by her always talking. Needing space to retreat into his own world, he had adopted *elective mutism*[1] as a means of coping.

Let us summarise the differences more specifically. Unlike his mother, Joey's need to understand *why*, and always *before* accepting any facts as facts, was highlighted by his strong personal preference for looking at the bigger picture. That complex way of reflecting on everything was clearly not Sondra's usual mode of functioning. For his mother, reality was never in dispute; she held a black-and-white stance on most issues, and no colour variations to be contemplated. After there had been valuable reflection and time spent with Sondra and her son, a good relationship eventually evolved that showed how love combined with understanding could nourish a developing young man. The likely alternative would have seen Joey and his mother becoming another tragic case of two warring or mismatched ships passing in the night: unable to relate through an *apparent* lack of care, but really due to a lack of seeing and understanding their differences.

After I built rapport with Joey, it was wonderful finally to engage in conversation with this capable young boy. On helping him understand his own needs and how these were different from his mother *and* from many others around him at school, it was so good to see his positive responses to now feeling he was understood. In time, this allowed Joey to realise more of his potentials with greater self-confidence. He could even enjoy his differentness.

With Sondra also now more cognisant of their very different ways of thinking, the new understanding offered a means of improved relationship potentials. Previously she had perceived others being different as potentially oppositional to her. This new understanding took away much of what had maintained her assumptions: that others disliked, rejected her, were nasty or selfish. This feeling of personal rejection is all too often associated with feeling different from others and not being understood.

Developing respectful ways for them to relate meant a growing improvement in Joey's capacity to enjoy life, rather than feeling constantly frustrated by his mother and her unrealistic expectations of him. From time to time separate sessions with Sondra were organised, as needed. This included encouraging her in ways that would assist Joey to become less introverted, at least with her and his teacher at school. Sondra also came to appreciate how her own more factual, "realist-constrained" personality typically at times had erupted when she expected him to be like her! Sondra and Joey were consequently able to anticipate potential hiccups when reminders of previous and unrealistic expectations of each other were suddenly reawakened.

Repetition needed to replace old habits

Learning to understand doesn't naturally or immediately produce acceptance or know-how, so their attempts to acquire new skills were monitored over several months. In this way, both mother and son had an outlet for expressing unmet needs with an outsider, helping each of them to better understand and accept their differences. At the same time, these sessions created important adjustment opportunities to clear the relationship airways again!

Personality-type research in psychology is built on a rigorous research framework, involving principles of psychometric validation[2] where the constructs can be seen to have an objective, neurologically related basis. This means that the constructs are not simply fanciful and abstract such as palmistry, numerology, or reading tea leaves, but evidence-based, with robust well-defined categories of individual differences. Much research has related these constructs to personal development, differing needs, differing ways of knowing and understanding, and importantly contribute much to mental health and adjustment. As such, they provide an exceptionally helpful means in counselling for better self-understanding and self-acceptance.

The WOT questionnaire

So, you may be asking: what do we mean by the terms Idea-ist and Realist, illustrated by the WOT questionnaire? Important research at Monash and Melbourne University into differences in ways of thinking (in which we were involved) has demonstrated that Idea-ist and Realist both refer to two contrasting Ways of Thinking captured by the WOT Inventory. This inventory is available for completion anonymously, giving self-reports online that highlight important individual differences.

Completing it online will hopefully not only be enjoyable but give you an understanding of these terms for yourself. See footnote for links to free version.[3]

Joey and Sondra were each strongly one-sided. With each the opposite of the other, until the differences were explained, understood, and accepted, neither appreciated the other's very differing needs, and consequently they regularly frustrated each other. This created considerable social anxiety for Joey, a boy still in the process of developing his identity.

While more minor differences may not be as frustrating as in this example, they can still create difficulties. Alternatively, when two individuals are attracted to each other simply because they both strongly seem to have the same way of thinking and feeling, they may miss out on the very possible benefits that being different can bring when dealing with the challenges life brings. Jamie and Melissa's case will be revealed shortly.

Clearly in Joey and Sondra's case we see a significant innate and genetically driven component in the way that individuals think, which becomes more evident developmentally through childhood. Joey had completed the children's version of the WOT.[4]

> *Consider how you may be the same or different from significant others you know well. How does that impact your relationship with them?*

WOT and approach to counselling

Another of the clearest cases illustrating the importance of understanding differences in thinking was that of a senior police officer who presented with a drinking problem. His wife of 35 years had sent him along with an ultimatum: "Fix your drinking or I am leaving you."

Arthur had been in the Armed Forces, serving overseas prior to joining the police force after discharge. On the face of it, here was a person one might easily assume suffered ongoing PTSD (post-traumatic stress disorder) so typically had self-medicated with alcohol. As I started to explore his history, and especially as I sought to *explain* what I was thinking and why, his eyes glazed over more and more. In thinking about how to engage him, I pondered whether he was here only at his wife's and family's behest.

To try to move the session to an opportunity for him to identify what problem he acknowledged, I asked him one of the essential questions: "What do you hope to get out of the sessions?" He gave an immediate, concise, and straight answer. He fully agreed with his wife that his drinking was out of control, and he needed to gain control over it. That was why he was here. His quick response provided the direct and practical statement that revealed his style of thinking: "I don't have to understand *why* I need to drink so much. I just need to get control."

One way of telling the difference between Realist and Idea-ist (not to be confused with *idealist*) is that the Realist typically wants to get on and do, while the Idea-ist needs to understand before they can do. Arthur's comment suggested that digging into the past, seeking to explain where he was at now, could be counterproductive. After a quick review of his WOT questionnaire, I decided to push forward, do as he asked, mindful that we could always move back to his history for a better understanding if needed.

Patterns of thinking affect behavioural habits

Elements of depression are inevitably a factor in such cases. Together we set up a programme around regular exercise (he had become largely desk-bound in his job). We talked about his drinking as a bad habit rather than an addiction. Having acknowledged the behavioural precursors, we set up a straightforward behavioural management programme based on *operant conditioning* principles. Here, experiencing the impulse to get a drink became instead a signal to do something else that was satisfying. This included going for a jog, or collaborating with his wife, and, to her delight, this even included asking how her day was going! Arthur had become somewhat of a workaholic, so he agreed to curtail work to reasonable hours to allow time to take up some relaxing and social activities.

Excellent satisfying progress over three months was confirmed in a review session twelve months later. Three factors stood out. The first was Arthur's sense of ownership of his problem, taking responsibility that also involved honesty and determination, in contrast to many addiction cases marked by self-deception and denial. Secondly, there was the supportive role of his wife and family, with reports of welcome relationship benefits. And thirdly, Arthur's natural orientation was to focus on doing. As a Realist, he now understood his expressed and obvious aversion to spending much time on personal reflection and also his lack of interest in meditational-type activities.

Another case already mentioned in Chapter 10 may help explain the efficacy of knowing personality type. You remember young Tim, and his focus on hand washing, which had generalised into an OCD compunction on many things. One of the best tools that helped his mother understand Tim was in knowing his personal profile – for example, his creative focus on ideas that meant he had always confused the facts. This was always more difficult for him because of his need to *understand* before he could *do*. These factors alone made much sense to them both, and contributed to their relief about his having a permanent mental illness that he would never be rid of. But Tim did need to manage his extreme scores, and, as it were, develop his left hand better!

Idea-ists: indecision lacking realistic insights

Jamie and Melissa were a couple who came for counselling because they could not decide about when to start having children; in fact, they were uncertain as to whether they ever wanted any children. Whenever the topic arose, they would experience a classical *approach-avoidance conflict.* No sooner would there be the suggestion that it might be time to start a family than all the associated encumbrances and the great responsibilities would surface yet again. As soon as they started talking about either postponing having a family or making a definite decision to not have one, both would feel so disappointed that the yearning for children would arise yet again. They had been together for nine years, and they told me this issue had been a constant for the last eight, and now, in their own words, was "getting louder, probably with a consciousness of the clock ticking".

Both were secondary school teachers: Jamie teaching fine arts and Melissa teaching humanities, history and literature. I asked them how they decided on things generally and the answer was that they would talk and talk, and think of many options, often creative and alternative, and then often not decide. It quickly became clear that both loved exploring ideas and possibilities, sharing them, imagining them, but then the next day there were new options to dream about. They recognised the pattern: it seemed that an idea or the dream was enough, as if it had already been experienced!

Jamie quickly gave an example. A few months before, with long service soon to be upon them both, they excitedly started planning an overseas trip. He wanted to go to Italy and France, and Melissa to Germany and the United Kingdom. They had trawled the internet and collected a range of brochures from the local travel agent. They had been quite excited with all they had learned, but then, after about a month, the interest waned. It was, Melissa said, as if they had already been and seen, and the thinking now was that they would rather stay at home where Jamie could sculpt and paint, and she could "veg out in a comfy chair reading some of the books" she had piled up!

Now that they were not going, they occasionally would say to the other, "wouldn't it have been fun!" As for taking up the long service leave, well, even that, too, had been shelved!

Both Jamie and Melissa enjoyed thinking and talking about ideas together. However, the doing was another matter. Further discussion revealed that they had developed loads of plans, like doing up the house, with wonderful designs for the garden. Inevitably they would think of alternatives, always wondering if there was a yet better plan and never really getting on to implementing any of them. Meanwhile, as they laughingly told me, there were a couple of leaks in the roof, in part caused by gutters overflowing because of pine needles from a huge tree in the front garden. Big ideas grew about the place of the pine tree in any future garden design, so yes, nothing changed.

I surmised: here was a delightful couple who clearly loved playing with ideas, including philosophising. *Both* being strong Idea-ists however meant that neither would bring an idea to fruition. To probe the idea that the reality of the practicalities of having young children might be problematic, I asked them what they feared most in having children. Melissa said she didn't know, but how she could cope with a helpless baby whom she could not talk to seemed to be her biggest worry. Jamie agreed, suggesting that the helpless baby phase actually frightened him too. On the other hand, he thought he would really look forward to when the child would be old enough to make stuff with him in his studio – but that would take years!

Idea-ists can often have loads of alternative ideas but then avoid making a balanced practical assessment and the plan to complete. What stands out at any one moment is whatever is front and centre. To check this out, I asked them how they had decided to marry. They both laughed before Jamie explained. One of Melissa's old flames, to her sorrow, had broken off with her, but then had broken off with his *new* girlfriend and returned to Melissa, wanting to resume their relationship. Melissa had told Jamie – whom she by then was dating – that she didn't know what to do: she cared for both the old flame and the new!

Distressed, Jamie had talked with a couple of friends who suggested the only way out of months of uncertainty was to get Melissa to make a decision, a commitment once and for all: he should test the waters by asking her to marry him. I turned to Melissa to ask how she came to decide to accept the proposal. She laughed, claiming he took advantage of her romantic side! Taking her out to a romantic dinner, he produced an engagement ring he had designed. How could she say "no" to that? Any potential alternatives were far out of mind, and once she had said "yes", she was never one to go back on her word. At that, Jamie looked somewhat sheepish but was reassured by Melissa then sensitively adding that, now after nine years, she knew it was one of the best decisions she'd ever made.

Making decisions: pros and cons

This narrative captures the anatomy of one couple's frustrating decision-making processes: too many viable alternative ideas, and no practical means of deciding between seeming equally attractive alternatives. They needed an objective way of weighing up. Had they ever written down the pros and cons of various options? To my surprise, no; deciding was always simply in their heads. Now, we know that Idea-ists can have many ideas, and keeping them all "up in the air" makes a balanced decision an almost impossible juggling act. But in terms of the marriage proposal, there was a clue: by being distracted by the emotion that overshadowed any Idea-ism, the couple could make the decision. A sound principle became evident for them: don't look back, live with what you have decided, and get on with life; don't ponder if it was the best decision.

We returned to their decision about having children. The couple were asked to write up a list of pros and cons, consider ways of mitigating/coping with any cons, and then weight each pro and con, coming out with a score. Having done that, they were then to set a commitment deadline for a conclusive decision. With a new understanding of their thinking styles, they started applying the newly learned decision-making process to other projects in their lives.

A couple of years later I met Melissa in the supermarket and, over a brief chat, she reflected on the past: Jamie always had his studio in which to create whatever he liked, but she had become somewhat of a couch potato, procrastinating about nearly every potential project. But now, she had developed a way of closing off a decision for action and prioritising, to make it happen. In fact, the childless future had been clearly dismissed, as was happily shown in her pushing a pram! She was no longer constantly frustrated by a lack of understanding herself, and by her typical long-held indecisiveness.

Although our personal way of thinking can be thought of as largely determined by our genes, our being aware of our natural inclination can also make us less likely to be overwhelmed by it. It can also mean, like many things in which we find an inherent weakness, we *can* learn to develop a less one-sided way of thinking. As mentioned earlier, Jung had reflected on this need – often only acknowledged at mid-life, and considered a luxury but worth exploring – to broaden individual coping strategies, growing the underdeveloped side of our personalities. This process can enrich us as individuals, but also can enable a greater appreciation of others' capacities and abilities – with the result that complementarity is understood, rather than seen as and felt to be a threat.

REFLECTIVE EXERCISES

If or when you have completed the WOT, take time to consider:

- Do you have a clearer understanding of how your thinking is different from or similar to others? How does this affect the way you feel about that?
- Do the explanations and feedback about the Idea-ist and Realist profiles make sense to you?

- Decide if you are strongly one way or the other, or perhaps somewhere in the middle; explaining this to a friend may be a great talking point!
- Can you or do you already use both ways of thinking, depending on the context?
- Is there a *cost* in using your less preferred thinking style? Does this perhaps cause you to reflect on the personal cost when having to use your Ideal or Expected Self instead of your Real Self?

It is important to understand that none of us tends to be exclusively either one or the opposite polarity on a disposition, but rather that one is preferred more strongly over the other, providing balance.

This is rather like being dominantly right- or left-handed: we still need to find the non-dominant hand as flexible and as adaptable as possible!

Notes

1 Elective mutism, now referred to as selective mutism, is sometimes recognised as a means of coping with social anxiety. Anxiety can be associated with perceptions of reality. There are numerous good resources explaining selective mutism on the internet.
2 Construct validation is an essential science for providing robust constructs often with associated measures, thereby facilitating evidence-based psychological practice. Wide-ranging scholarly debate has advanced the science. For an excellent coverage see K Slaney, *Validating Psychological Constructs: Historical, Philosophical, and Practical Dimensions* (London, Palgrave MacMillan, 2017).
3 The general information website for adolescents or older of the WOT is: www.waysofthinking.org. The link to specifically *taking* the WOT is: www.waysofthinking.org/take.
4 The plan is to develop a WOT-C version, to become available online within the next couple of years, making it available for any child under the guidance of an informed parent or counsellor.

Chapter 14

Identity grounded in self-acceptance

In this chapter we build on previous two chapters that highlighted individual differences in how dispositions impact our behaviours, and importantly note how others often react to these distinctive characteristics. Here we further consider individual differences as related to our identity. An understanding of our identity often has important ramifications on those around us. Understanding of self involves recognition of feelings and beliefs that often belie a reality about ourselves that really demands an answer to the puzzling question: who am I? Further questions repeatedly revolve around an understanding of the internal conflict created by unconscious demands on defining expectations of who we are: the Real Self (who I really and naturally am, largely driven by my innate traits, my personality and abilities), the Ideal Self (who I aspire to be – my ideals and values), and the Expected Self (others' expectations of who I should be – social pressure). Resolutions made about any tensions between these three selves can also be shown to benefit relationships, making decisions about our choices more realistically satisfying when living or working with others. Before getting down to case exemplars, there is a need to understand identity, which involves considering its formation: a multiplicity of cogent influences that are acknowledged within limits and focus.

Beyond personality: greater self-understanding

You must have heard someone exclaim using the term "personality" in a popular sense– "Oh, they are such great personalities – great fun to be with". Or, after watching a show, comments like, "Such a mix of personalities – a bit confusing – couldn't get the gist of the plot, all too complex!" You may also have noticed how commonly the notion of what personality means relates to liking or not liking a person or their behaviours! We explored the complex and psychological nature of personality in Chapters 12 and 13. Whichever way you look at it, after reading those chapters we can agree that we each have a personality, a persona that is unique.

DOI: 10.4324/9781003474746-14

> *Many individuals lack any real understanding of themselves, their personality, and who they really are, which can make it equally difficult for them to be known and appreciated by others.*

Questionnaires that ask: who am I really?

Hopefully by now *you* will have completed one of the inventories discussed in the previous chapters, or one of the many personality questionnaires readily available. In moving on to the ubiquitous question of identity, we hope you have enjoyed positive identification of important and valued factors about your own unique personality, with an understanding that may also have contributed to your identity. Discovering your preferred dispositions can be a wonderful contribution to a wholesome sense of identity: "This is me, and I'm really glad to be *me*!" Regardless of whether you are like me, a practical doer to whom details are important, or like my important other, a strong intuitive ideas thinker who more values the big picture and *understanding*, we can learn to appreciate each other's uniqueness. As differently oriented and gifted individuals, we can appreciate that others may more naturally do what we can't do – and vice versa!

If perchance your results from any such a questionnaire have left you somewhat confused or questioning yourself, a discussion with others who know you well may offer an explanation – either about how you answered questions, or whether the real you is still evolving.

If you have not yet looked specifically at your own personality profile, hopefully it is not because the previous chapters have failed to waylay any concerns that may have been holding you back from exploring your dispositions. If so, let us encourage you: whenever we have run workshops or given feedback to individuals, we are always surprised to find how affirming those descriptors usually are when properly understood. Such understanding is in part reported in the case examples we have given. In short, we consider that any trustworthy understanding should be empowering and benefit anyone in any people-helping role. Remember the point made in the previous chapters, that personality inventories – unlike measures of ability (next, in Chapter 15) which aim to clarify your various capabilities – look at valid and reliable descriptors (or factors) of *preferred* characteristics about how individuals operate. These demonstrate that we actually do hold many of these in common with at least some other humans.

Remember also if you are concerned about being boxed, any report of your dispositional personality profile should not be confining. Rather, you may be alerted to things about yourself that you may benefit from acknowledging and understanding – for example, where it leads to working on some previously underdeveloped part of your personhood should make you feel a more rounded, complete and whole.[1] By realistically understanding our profile, our identity as a person who is worth knowing is inevitably enhanced. Having happily accepted that picture, we are presented with a stronger sense of self, of our identity, both reaffirming and indisputable, and, in that, empowering. Building on such an understanding of self, we move on to unpack implications about identity.

Modern take on what identity involves

An explanation of identity has often simplistically considered only obvious personal attributes such as physical and behavioural traits, with perhaps a strong acceptance of your name, eye colour, skin colour, and even fingerprints, all once understood from within one's stable cultural or tribal norms and folkways, often handed down over generations.

Beside these factors and the dispositions that we have been considering, let us consider what other significant factors impact on identity formation.

Culture itself is seen to impact identity. With international travel and migration has come a broader exposure to a wider range of differing cultures. The plurality inherent in multiculturalism is increasingly raising many questions, some that provide conflicting answers that reflect new heterogeneous social orders. Understanding the close relationship between belonging and identity offers some insight into how identity formation is no longer a simple matter of accepting a set of unambiguous community values.

Where there is increased wealth, consumerism, and marketing in the context of secularisation life and identity have become even more seen as being about having a choice. The belief has emerged that all that determines identity is fluid, a *dynamic* view of identity previously not thought possible.

Challenges to sexual identity, once historically considered as fixed, discrete, and an indicator of expected roles and behaviour, have increasingly taken centre stage following on from the sexual revolution of the 20th century. For many, no longer is gender identification considered to be defined by the physical genital characteristics one is born with. Others maintain varying cultural and religion-based views. A potpourri of differing opinions, many often subjective and strongly held, are complicated and influenced by the ubiquitous never-ending nature/nurture debate. Complex sexual identity issues become further convoluted by the need to identify with certain groups, with the enormous pressure created by an individual's need to belong currently being one potent social factor.

Without entering into a debate as to what is negotiable and what is not, how do we approach the core understandings needed in practice for treading effectively through the fraught identity minefield?

The need to belong

We return to the iterative relationship between identity and belonging. A sense of belonging has long been an accepted personal essential that results from giving and receiving acceptance, respect, and love.[2] Though understood by some as a common motivation for self-actualisation, the desire to belong is intuitively and universally accepted as a basic human need associated with our identity. Both research and lived experiences demonstrate the negative effects suffered by the person who is seriously restricted in meeting this powerful and basic need for belonging.

For some, it embraces a deep-seated need for freedom of choice about their individuality. Identity for these individuals lies in finding themselves in their autonomy and independence. For others, a stronger need exists in the context of wanting connection, and for them identity is typically determined by relationships and connection. Such different preferences are inevitably also impacted by cultural and religious values. With increasing multiculturalism, this complexity presents societal challenges, such as how we accept and live peaceably with our obvious differences, not least in our conflicting values, all conflicts that demand understanding and attention.

Issues that could be included

There are many identified issues that impact an individual's validating their own personal identity. Beyond the brief understanding articulated above, this book does not aim to cover and debate the plethora of controversial underlying values and issues that surround identity formation. That would require a volume on its own. If you need some clarification, we hope you will research these issues well.

Suffice to say, healthy identity formation is clearly needed for well-being. There is currently a global recognition of problems associated with gender aspects of identity formation that have seen governments from differing countries pass conflicting legislation. Debates rage even within countries. The resolutions of many associated issues are impossible to achieve with satisfaction for all. Meanwhile, individuals still need loving support while working through their identity, in identity formation, and in overcoming any developmental arrest. So the focus here will be on ways of effectively supporting and counselling, respecting clients and their values, not on any debate of assumptions.

> *Our own personal views may often differ dramatically from each other as carers, so they will most certainly differ from those of many clients and their respective agendas. Throw into that the complexities of cultures that make new demands, parents having their own opinions, or a child's undeveloped questions needing to be answered well and not just simply gratified! We must be serious about really listening, hearing the many and varied views, and maintaining an unconditional positive regard before deciding to offer our objectively considered perspectives. It is so important to know our own limitations and expertise about the issues involved, to prevent us taking unnecessary responsibility for approving or criticising others for their actions.*

I will just share two exemplars from some years ago, as a brief commentary only on the broader context of identity that is posed by gender/sexuality contentions.

Sexual and gender identity

The first case was an older lady, Maria, concerned about an upcoming visit by her adult daughter from overseas. Jodie had joined a lesbian group in London, enjoying her freedoms without the restrictions of her previous culture and family. Maria had not told her husband this, knowing that because of his age and cultural background he would be very upset. Maria however wanted Jodie to understand her deep concerns about what would happen to the family should Jodie's perceived "aberrant behaviour" be shared with her unwell father. Maria wanted me to explain this to Jodie. She also had another agenda: that Jodie should become convinced that what she was doing was wrong!

Before Jodie's return, an appointment was made with Maria, after I had explained I was happy only with the first request, in order to help spare Maria much distress at home. Jodie's mother also gradually appreciated being given some insights into an adult child's right to make their own decision about their sexual preferences.

The session with Jodie was quite positively received, with Jodie openly sharing some reasons she believed had led to her decision against heterosexual relationships, one importantly that reflected on her lack of attachment to her father. Jodie also made it clear that she was of the view that she had choice in these matters. Clearly it was important for Jodie to ally herself with her "London tribe of women", so she was happy to maintain that alliance for now – though she granted the possibility that she could change, or alternatively, might even have a sex change operation!

In answer to carefully worded open-ended questions, Jodie spoke willingly but briefly about potential repercussions, like eventually perhaps wanting to have a child, but for now she was determined to just enjoy the moment. However, she did agree that it was kinder to keep her present orientations and inherent values conflict from her father, to prevent a potential drama and distress for the people she loved while home in Australia. She was pleased to have at least been alerted to her father's serious ill-health, and equally relieved that her adult decisions were not likely to destroy relationships at home. Some issues were explored respectfully, but my task was done.

Having seen Jodie off, Maria attended once more, reassured that her daughter had not totally lost her childhood values of caring for others. Though disappointed by Jodie's determination to retain her current *sexual* identity, Maria lived with her own aspirations for Jodie, and it was not my prerogative to dissolve them.

The second person who comes to mind attended for help in order to be able to reveal to others that she was shortly to undergo "a sex change operation". She had already commenced hormone treatment, evidenced by facial hair that matched her more masculine hairstyle. Felicity had immediately indicated to me she did *not* need or want any advice about changing her decision but, rather, she wanted to know how best to alert her children to what her next step would entail.

Question: how would you approach this problem? Would you feel a need to accrue more information about the ensuring medical intervention?

Perhaps you already recognise that there may be other matters like attachments that need to be explored.

Communications between us needed to focus on Felicity's explicit request, which naturally allowed me to ask for family details. I needed to know how she thought each of her children might react. But it became clear that another issue was important, as she talked about her family of origin, admitting she had never felt accepted as a girl. Her parents were always saying they had wanted a boy! In trying to please, she had continued their pattern by dressing herself as a boy, though said that, with her imaginative artistic mind, she often struggled with the inner conflict aroused in her around her own identity. She'd happily married quite young but until recently had never acknowledged how she really felt about herself, and who she was. As a child, asking such questions about herself was never considered important enough to be given much thought. Communications at home had always been limited.

Her husband of some twenty years had accepted Felicity's recent activities in now questioning who she was, which included cross-dressing at home, though he had made it clear he didn't want his friends to know – so life had to just go on as it had in the past. Everyone already thought of Felicity as an "arty tomboy" – but interestingly, she reported no expectations or disappointment expressed from her friends about any perceived lack of femininity. The sharing of these details allowed me to ask about her personal self-acceptance. Questions like how much did her self-doubt rest in continual childhood disapprovals, experiences that had made her feel worthless or unacceptable?

Honest answers revealed a childhood that was far from happy. Her artistic strengths were seen as ridiculous, so no encouragement was given to affirm her as an individual with talents, which in turn impacted her beliefs about her intelligence and gave her equally negative feelings about her identity. Type-casting had been even more of an issue, making the sensitive and introverted Felicity increasingly concerned about what others thought of her, which became convoluted into a confused sexual identity: her dress codes suggesting she was not a "normal" female. You can hear her self-doubts, and her expressed grief and sadness about an upbringing that had never properly been confronted, let alone resolved.

The end of her story? Well, many questions were posed that Felicity needed to answer realistically – for example, who would the teenage children see her to be, as a full-on male? Her response of "Oh, a favourite uncle, I guess" was a sure indicator of her lack of insight into the potential reality of future relationships. But in spite of such alerts, including that her family might well reject her when her changed sexual orientation became known more publicly, Felicity did inform her children, and what seemed inevitable did happen. Her husband took the children – he angrily declared he was not gay, so had no intention of being forced to look like he was.

Many months later, I again met with Felicity; she had clearly reversed her decision, acknowledging the pain of losing her family. And by finally confronting past issues, she admitted to now developing a healthier self-acceptance, so that the children eventually were again able to see her as their mother. Felicity indicated a growing appreciation of her uniqueness, and that her natural artistic abilities/interests needed no stereotypical confirmation by any sexual or gender orientation.

What is your response?

Observing the complex decisions our society is currently dealing with in regard to gender issues, few right/wrong answers are found to be acceptable by all.

This is particularly apparent within the identity issues surrounding LGBTI+ and similar transgender/non-binary issues, creating enormous problems of identity for our young people. The question for many remains difficult when presented as a matter of choice. Laws are constantly being re-evaluated. And where children had been apportioned life-changing physiological solutions, some – now as hurting maturing adults – are refuting decisions made on their behalf, deemed inappropriate at least, with others demanding that those they regard as responsible be held accountable.

Regardless of whether or not you are responsible for finding answers that confront these mammoth confusions, make sure that your attitudes are clear and well-based in facts, not just opinions that will change with the winds that blow hardest! Such demands of "freedom to be who I want to be" are often heard from a small but powerful group or tribe, intent on influencing others, needing others to join them, with little concern for the longer effect on the individual, let alone on society in general. Such freedoms seem to suggest wishful thinking often associated with immaturity, wanting youthful experimentation, without thoughtful knowledge of repercussions or consequences. Much like the problems facing the unrestricted licensing of young drivers to drive fast cars; lack of experience and possibly hormonal upheaval leading to risk-taking is common, until age provides the missing knowledge and wisdom that can modify their behaviour.

Remain caring of the individuals being dragged into these dilemmas at an increasingly young age. But be unapologetic and honest in your own appraisal of the realities associated with choices they may make. Much wisdom[3] is needed if we are to provide good alternative insights, to assist individuals strained by confusions. All too often it seems as if human sexual identity is simply something to be amorally open to being exploited, rather than understood and valued, both for the individual and for the benefit of the community.

Reflection time on identity

Personal question: on what does your identity depend?

Does your profession and its title provide your main or perhaps your only identity? Is it your family? Or maybe how well you are known or liked? Does your identity depend on your sexual orientation?

What would you write, if asked to write your own obituary? As an individual, how would you like others to remember you?

Many of our beliefs, particularly about ourselves, and the important values we hold precious form a huge part of our identity. Yet the notion of belonging seems to have taken pride of place today. Our need for acceptance and connection means we often seek to be among similarly thinking and behaving people, who share the same beliefs and values: our tribe. However, regardless of age, a strong individual need remains: to find a satisfying self-acceptance that provides a confidence in one's identity.

Who am I?

With a brief glance back to Chapter 9 you will find reference to Viktor Frankl,[4] and his search for the meaning of life. Another gem from his memoir points to the principle that we have found so importantly connected to good relationships, one that asks the following questions in this order:

"Who am I?", "Where am I going?", and then "Who will go with me?"

Finding a deep and meaningful answer to the first question requires serious reflection, which can be especially difficult if we have not grown up in a loving environment, not made to feel comfortable in our own skin. The negative flow-on effect of a lack of valued attachment to our parents of course also impacts on future relationships, so that others will not know who we are either. This can lead to us *performing* as if our self-belief is not in question, and all manner of compensatory behaviours[5] can be observed, and without an apparent rationale. Carl Jung,[6] the psychiatrist/psychotherapist active almost one hundred years ago, also understood this self-knowledge confusion experienced by many of his clients, who well into their middle years were still trying to find themselves. In the uncovering of the unknown dimensions of the "self" previously left undeveloped, a personal understanding and acceptance of that whole self could then be appreciated.

Self-knowledge that satisfies

When people discover a deeper insight into who they really are, when their individual inclinations and individuality are clearly known, they often express surprise, then relief. Recall here Sheryll (Chapter 10), who, after a disturbing drug reaction, had faced potential and predicted mental illness, until learning that her vulnerabilities related to her personal tendency to depend on others for approval. Self-doubt had previously thwarted her efforts to believe in herself, while feeling like a square peg in a round hole!

Another such person comes to mind: Tony, an electrician who was sick of the "boring life" he had run with for many years, feeling frustrated in the jobs he had simply taken on for money, without any enjoyment or personal satisfaction. Questioned about what it was like growing up, he reported much of the same dissatisfaction. Little money in his migrant family meant that he was expected to leave school quite young, to get a practical job. He admitted he never really thought of himself as intelligent, and had married the girl next door, who equally seemed "accepting of her lot in life".

Rather than continuing to be frustrated, his wife Pippa had encouraged Tony to see someone, to get help with his moodiness. Latterly he'd even found getting out of bed quite difficult. Tony questioned me about how he would cope if this deadly depressing future remained unchanged.

An initial approach enabled us to consider what miniscule possibilities he might uncover if we looked at his earlier preferences – first recalling what at primary school he had loved doing. Drawing and painting had been his great enjoyment back then. So again with his wife's encouragement, he started a new hobby: making wooden toys for his young children, with a great sense of personal pride and satisfaction.

My Real, my Ideal, or my Expected Self?

Too often, the question of "who am I" is confusing, particularly if we are unaware of the internal conflict that can exist between our three selves.

The diagram below may help explain what sometimes causes some intra-personal or internal tensions, making self-knowledge confusing, both difficult to understand and manage.

Identity formation

Development of individual identity is seen to begin at birth, initially influenced by various factors such as family and friends. Each individual is born with

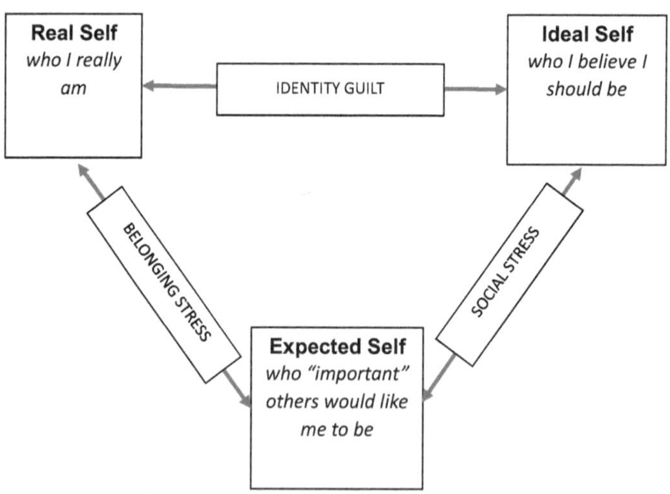

Figure 14.1 Intra-personal tensions between Real, Ideal, and Expected Self-perceptions

an incredible and innate set of personality characteristics, capacities, and abilities, forming an identity wonderfully linked to their genes. Increasingly as self-consciousness develops, self-perceptions receive affirmation and approval (or not), as external social influences create important contributions that impact an individual's sense of self.

Sadly, many of these influences can distort that original innocent identity of self to such a degree that "finding oneself" becomes a lifetime endeavour. Think again to young Tim in Chapter 10 – developing his healthy sense of self might have remained unknown, except for his growing knowledge of self, enabled by truthful communications, psychological insights, and affirmations through appropriate assessments.[7]

Or remember Sheryll, also Chapter 10, whose identity may have been permanently confused by peer pressure, depriving her of a clear trajectory for a positive development of her identity. Constructive change, brought on by a traumatic event (drug taking), created a personal rethink moment of lasting import.

Of course, there will be times when our Real Self needs to consider other possible formative pressures, identified as the Expected Self and/or Ideal Self. The value of knowing these different selves can indeed empower further positive growth to our identity, providing *choices* in challenging situations. Circumstances such as those mentioned throughout earlier chapters provide examples, like being a parent of a rebellious teenager. Concern for a difficult child (see Joan with her teenage daughter, Chapter 4) may demand that a personal preference and desire for control be put aside, choosing to use an *Ideal* Self that behaves more honourably, less impatiently than what a more *Real* Self would do!

Alternatively, in the case of someone who has been brought up to do only what they *feel* like doing, with no reference to caring about others, the Real Self has not learned to modify a natural self-centredness that can alienate. This means that a wiser, more socially aware self does not develop, or at least is delayed. Consequently, we can reflect on the spoilt child, for whom maturation into a well-grounded individual becomes difficult. The self-centred identity usually experiences considerable difficulty in making and maintaining relationships with others who do not understand or accept the value of self-centredness!

Effect on parenting style

I am reminded of several parents who presented with such children, and yet who had not realised what personal issues of their own had impacted their parenting styles. Some had unconsciously contributed to the development of their "out of control" spoilt child. You will see this in Chapter 18 (Caring for the Carer) in the case of Vera, a busy mother struggling to meet the demands of her Expected

Self, when trying also to care for her frail mother. As a response to how much was *expected* of her while growing up, Vera had really lost sight of her Real Self, meaning that without reflection, she had been driven to overcompensate for her children, as a reaction to her own past. Her Ideal Self had simply over-ridden her own personal needs, thinking that she should always behave as an ideal mother would.

Perhaps there is enough here to allow you to reflect on how you appreciate knowing *about* the differences between these three selves. Reflect back on the examples given in Chapter 13: Ways of Thinking, as an appreciation of how the way we think actually helps to validate our identity. Reflection here may help you consider how any conflict between our three selves might need to be minimised.

> *When we utterly accept who we are, we can still make choices about how much we allow our* ***Ideal*** *self or our* ***Expected*** *self to dominate our* ***Real*** *self. The whole or complete self is available – so long as we make wise choices!*

Accepting our true identity is more possible when we feel comfortable in our own skin, believing we are uniquely different, an individual with foibles and strengths who is yet lovable and capable of love. This infers that we do not *need* to be like others, nor should we suffer from the stress imposed by an unrealistic Ideal self, or be driven by what others expect us to be, simply to belong.

You may have seen a recent wonderful example of this, provided by Australia's current cricket captain, Pat Cummins.[8] He confronted criticisms with the statement "I know who I am . . . my friends and family know who I am" – saying that he didn't have to pander to a crowd mentality or powerful minority. What a great acknowledgment of the wisdom and blessing of confidently and humbly knowing who you are. The flow-on effect comes next!

Where am I going?

When Tony (the electrician mentioned above) was trying to grasp who he really was, he completed a brief personality questionnaire,[9] and agreed to openly discuss at home what this revealed about his natural traits and preferences. Again, with his wife's encouragement, Tony initiated several weekly sessions to intensely rethink who he was, and what he really enjoyed doing. Fortunately, Tony had been a good electrician and had earned a substantial income. This process of self-discovery gave him obvious relief: as he was still only 36, there was time to think beyond his perceived constraining dark "forever-box" of an unsatisfied electrician!

Tony is a good example of potential changes a person can make, particularly with a right self-assessment, and a clearer understanding of one's natural abilities. His intellectual abilities, previously considered to be just average, were then assessed. It was important that he used this opportunity to also rethink his future, making enquiries about new career courses he might do, even if only in the evenings, until his pathway ahead was more than simply dreaming. See more on abilities in Chapter 15.

Clarity through understanding natural interests and abilities

Small but well-hidden dreams were activated: doing an art project, using his creative drawing abilities, as well as his love of working with wood. It was heart-warming when, sometime later, he brought in one of his beautifully crafted wood carvings, completed during an art class.

There were additional benefits from accepting then exploring his unique identity. The first one provided greater personal clarity: looking forward to choosing the best career path for a more satisfying life journey, exploiting natural talents and interests and the creativity that flowed from these. The second question – where am I going? – then became something not nearly so daunting.

> *A strong characteristic of self-acceptance is to be able to love others as you love/accept yourself, without the need to be defensive, jealous, or indeed a need to justify yourself.*

Such self-acceptance also gives a truly wonderful release: to confidently hold some values or beliefs as precious, though they may be quite different from those around you. An honest self-knowledge enables a more trustworthy understanding about where you would like to go, and creates a wonderful motivation, particularly as it merges with a *realistic* understanding of your ability to make that happen.

So we look at the third question associated with positive self-understanding:

Who's going with me?

When a satisfactory conclusion is made to the first two questions, even if only partially known, it becomes more plausible to consider a synergy with another person or other people who might journey with us. In Tony's case, though the decision of "who will go with me" was made many years before, he had always felt quite supported by his wife Pippa, almost like growing up together. She herself had recently begun her own journey to learn more about herself, prompted by lovingly watching her own children growing as individuals. Together Tony and Pippa were now more able to negotiate some of the changes each faced, with an unselfishness that made this commitment to a new start still quite daunting, yet also exciting.

Identity that benefits self and fellow travellers

The answer to this third question will apply equally to various situations. Whether as couples, partners in business, or as a team of people working together on a particular project, each relationship requires a respectful understanding and acceptance of each of the others. Such knowledge can maximise the potentials of various shared gifts. Goal setting also becomes more realistic, with the acknowledgement of both the strengths and the limitations of each individual involved.

In honestly becoming more aware of and accepting our limitations, we may realise what confusing elements may have been inherited or simply modelled ("I'm just like my Dad" or "I just copied what my dad did!"). Other behaviours and unrealistic self-perspectives can be identified as having been behaviours learnt along the way, when adapting to the demands expected of us.

Healthy self-reflection can also reveal any self-deprecation that may need another's perspective, some outside information about the "differentness" in our personal and preferred ways of thinking and behaving that otherwise remain hidden. Our personal identity, our innate characteristics, can sometimes be hidden from ourselves, which then becomes confusing for others. A trustworthy confidante may be a great first step.

An internal battle can be noted for a naturally left-handed child when forced to be a right-hander. This challenge is even more obvious in the person who tries hard to be someone s/he isn't. Deeper self-knowledge can create a greater understanding of why the apparent *mis*understandings about oneself have been allowed to control the choices one has made.

We hope you personally have reflected on your own identity – how grateful you will feel to be accepting of who you really are! When such knowledge is appreciated by the individual self, this understanding will also prove to be important to others with whom we interact.

REFLECTIVE EXERCISES

Do clarify any issues that may prevent you from being at home in your own skin. Share with an important other what may seem too difficult to tackle, to gain encouragement to find solutions that be satisfying to your Real Self.

Notes

1 Refer again to Jung, and the follow-up work of Myers and Briggs, from the mid-20th century.
2 See Maslow's Hierarchy of Needs, 1943.
3 See wisdom (Proverbs 4:6–8).
4 Victor Frankl, *Man's Search for Meaning*, originally published in 1946 in German; many editions are currently available.
5 In Compensatory Psychology a behavioural strategy seeks to cover weakness. Consider for example the psychology of Alfred Adler. There are many excellent references on the internet explaining his Theory of Personal Psychology and Individuality.
6 Wikipedia offers a good starting point of learning about the groundbreaking Jung.
7 For example, the Australian Psychological Society's College of Educational and Developmental Psychology specifically describes its focus as being a commitment to personal growth over the life span.
8 https://www.abc.net.au/news/2023-11-28/pat-cummins-criticisms-world-cup-victory-.
9 See the popular MBTI (Myers Briggs Type Indicator), WOT (in Chapter 13), as well as the Big Five Personality Measure. The Five Factor personality theories form a well-accepted and validated body of research which along with measuring instruments are readily available via the internet.

Chapter 15

Assessment of abilities and learning difficulties

Across the lifespan there are various periods when the abilities question comes to the fore. From the newborn whose obvious potential abilities are still undeveloped, through to the elderly, with reduced capabilities in specific areas, both cognitive and physical, while often still feeling like they did in their prime! Assessment of where such people are at can be quite challenging. Learning difficulties are often not identified early enough. In this chapter we review several people at different stages of life, to illustrate how a cognitive appraisal can facilitate understanding, along with its useful practical implications. Formal testing is not dismissed, but rapport and informal observations are seen as important, an integral part of any comprehensive assessment to provide significant validation and deeper understanding of abilities beyond test conclusions.

The Public Trustee

Charles limped in looking slightly dishevelled. He sat down heavily in the consulting room chair. He showed an air of something like resignation, despair, or frustration as he held out the doctor's referral.

> *"Please advise on 81-year-old Charles's competence for self-management and provide necessary counselling. His affairs are currently controlled by the Public Trustee following a fall while living alone at home when intoxicated. His home of 46 years is currently rented out and he lives in a hostel. He is becoming increasingly depressed. He comes in and continually asks to be given back charge of his own affairs, but the next-of-kin is his daughter, who Charles laments is forcefully intervening, trying to ensure maintenance of current arrangements. His solicitor has suggested referral for psychological assessment."*

DOI: 10.4324/9781003474746-15

Charles's answer as to what he wanted out of coming to see me was clear and direct: to get the Public Trustee out of his life and to get back into his own home. When I enquired as to what the problem was in being looked after by the Public Trustee and living in the hostel, he suggested I should try it, "to find out what it's like!" Had I failed to establish rapport by responding to him in the direct way he had spoken, I wondered? But then I had a sense that it was not time to ask about his feelings, but rather to turn his suggestion around, asking him to tell me what made the arrangement most frustrating *for him.*

His answer was short: he didn't have access to his money for playing the stock market, and they had sold all his shares and invested his money in a low interest rate deposit account! Now he could neither buy the wine he liked, nor cook and enjoy his favourite Italian food. This gave me a natural opportunity to start a conversation about wines, Italian food, and the stock market. I also asked him to explain what he saw as the best strategies for playing the share market. He was clearly up to date with what was going on, and his strategy was mainly to invest in stable shares, while also willing to "gamble on a small part of the market" which he compared with betting on the horses. I perceived he was aware that my interest was more than just learning from him and was quick to assure me that he never gambled without a reasonable assessment of the odds.

When I sensed we had established sufficient rapport, I moved on to ask him where these interests had come from, as a way of moving over to his history. He needed little prompting, telling me of his life as a financial journalist after initial training as an accountant. The storytelling was colourful to the point of entertaining. He was focused and the telling evidenced a life-long coping mechanism: a dark Australian sense of humour. He described his journalistic culture – the smoking and drinking that had gone along with his long hours exploring the deceptions within the financial world. His love of Italian food had developed from a stint writing about food and wine in his final couple of years when working freelance. I noted that while the story was colourful, it was detailed, down to earth, with little sense of poetic licence. It exuded his preferences as a Realist in terms of his thinking style. Without any doubt, he still had outstanding journalistic abilities.

I needed to probe him about his family and friends, and as I did so, he became quiet. I thought I had lost him. There was silence for a couple of minutes as he now sat slumped forward. Then, in a quietened voice, he told me of his wife who had died six years prior. But that, he said, is what happens in life: "take it on the chin." He did not want to talk about her, other than that she and his daughter had been "as thick as thieves": had always ganged up on him. As for friends, they no longer visited him since he had been in the hostel.

> *Recounting the past is one thing, but coping in the present may be quite a different matter. Social support and friendships make a significant contribution to coping for most people and never more so than as we age.*

At this point he made it clear that he wanted to get on with what he saw was the business of me finding him to be competent enough to manage his own affairs, including at home. I explained that I thought a comprehensive ability set of tests would be best, and he agreed. Again, his self-deprecating humour was shared, laughing about how much his drinking may have affected his brain and which parts.

I explained to Charles how ability testing and neuropsychology has come a long way from simple one-score IQ notions. In the last couple of decades research has produced a comprehensive model across the distinctly separate abilities that make up the overall IQ score. These distinct abilities are considered to be akin to the periodic table in Chemistry, and testing instruments have been developed to cover all the various areas.

While his processing speed was a little slow, his results showed no cognitive deficits: indeed, all his abilities were in what is considered the "gifted" range – of being over two standard deviations above the mean (average) for his age. Only one area was not exceptional: spatial abilities, which were still average for his age. Interestingly, even when all abilities are well above a disability level, such relative differences in abilities within a person can result in their feelings of having a disability. We will explore that more in the next example but before doing so, let us consider the outcomes.

Aware that Charles was cognitively competent despite years of heavy drinking, for the purposes of a report to the Public Trustee, I needed to ascertain his capacity for taking responsibility. My questions were therefore quite direct: did he consider himself an alcoholic, and if so, why was his alcoholism not sufficient reason for him to remain under the control of the Public Trustee?

His answers were clear. He did not see his heavy drinking as anyone else's problem but his own. He knew he could take himself back to Alcoholics Anonymous. He had always enjoyed drinking, yet still had been able to manage his financial and personal affairs. Under his present living arrangements, he could still arrange to drink heavily and was more likely to do so out of sheer boredom and frustration. It was a matter of being able to do the things he *loved* that made life worthwhile: cooking, having some old mates around to eat and drink with, and playing the stock market instead of sitting in a dingy hostel room, playing Sudoku and waiting for the next dish of tasteless mash!

To check out whether his claim to cooking was not something invented just to persuade me, I started a conversation about what he liked doing in cooking. It soon became clear that it was a deep passion of his; he had a discriminating palate fired by a great deal of creative experimentation.

The results were reported to the Public Trustee and left for them to weigh up whether to discharge. As predicted, his family resented his subsequent independence. A few months later, Charles dropped by to thank me, saying it was so good to have his life back again, even though sometimes he might not behave as his family thought he should!

Learning disabilities – the road narrows

In contrast to Charles, Annie was a nine-year-old in grade 4 who seemed capable yet continued to experience difficulties with spelling and reading, despite being put through several programmes such as reading recovery and also receiving personal tuition. The teachers at the school wondered whether her particular ethnic background, combined with ambitious successful professional parents, had set unrealistic expectations.

I suspected that this girl was experiencing significant differences between her various capabilities, confirmed by my running her through an appropriate ability test battery. Her responses during the assessment reflected the discouraged image she had formed of herself. Much of the testing needed to be presented as a game, and fully explained as we went through. Items are presented in a sequence increasing in difficulty to the point of failure across a few items determining an ability level. As soon as Annie failed any single item, she would want to give up, but responded well when it was explained to her that this was the aim, and that even with a genius, we would get to items such a person could not do.

The testing itself had an intrinsic therapeutic aim, that is, it was diagnostic rather than classificatory.

So, no rigid sticking to protocols to get some supposedly objective number. Rather, a relaxed discussion ran like a game, discussing what each sub-test was about, and indicating how well she was going as we went along. The process of working collaboratively developed important rapport and started to build her self-confidence. With her performance no longer strangled by her lack of confidence, this success effectively challenged her belief in thinking she was stupid. Then, when we came to the memory tests, we were able to laugh and joke as we found an explanation as to why reading and spelling was such a frustration for her.

How should we explain the implications to a near ten-year-old in a way that would allow her to develop a positive means of accommodation, to understand and apply all the information she would receive? After all, so often any obvious individual difference is seen as somehow pathological, in need of being treated or remediated.

> *Accommodation means acceptance, understanding, developing the means of coping with any frustrations or difficulties that arise.*

Testing showed that Annie had a relatively poor short-term memory (STM). STM in cognition is recognised as a specific capacity on which individuals differ of being able to hold a number of specific integers in mind and recall them almost immediately. STM plays an important role in reading. To help Annie understand, we talked of trying to fill a large bottle with a narrow, restricted opening: plenty of capacity but frustrating to get some stuff in. She understood, and so did her parents when I used the analogy of a four-lane highway going into a single lane for a bridge or roadworks. There is little that can be done to directly improve such a poor STM; however, there are some useful strategies. We talked about clumping numbers together when needing to recall them, say for making a phone call, or spending extra time repeatedly using flash cards based on the Dolch or Fry Word lists of frequently used words.

The impact of such understanding can be and in this case was quite profound. Annie now had a much more real sense of self. She no longer identified herself as "the [discouraged] girl who could not spell", but the "girl who was determined and persistent". Her parents' understanding enabled them to support Annie, with a positive affirming attitude that replaced their worry, confirmed her as a person, admired and encouraged not the least for her persistence. Thinking about her as lazy and distracted had been dispelled.

A 12-month check-up showed that Annie was thriving. No more school refusal. When I asked her how she felt about learning new words, she said she just pictured the small necked bottle and saw determination in getting the stuff in as a challenge, knowing that the more she persisted, the more she inevitably got it in.

> *Analogies and metaphors can be so powerful!*

A realistic expectation is such an important part of self-acceptance, and so essential for well-being. This is often made possible when a simple picture or story becomes the trigger for hope.

Learning difficulties: when there is no road

Another case reveals how learning difficulties can be ignored for too long. Arham was already in Year 12 and came in with his father. The reason for attending? He had difficulty navigating his way home from work experience: not just once or twice at the beginning but continuing to have problems after two weeks. In part, the problem was solved by giving Arham cards with written instructions. Now, however, the school had finally recommended he get help, suggesting it could be a long-term issue. They questioned whether he might have some sort of spatial problem.

If there was such a problem, I pondered how it had not manifested earlier. Asking about his family soon gave me an answer. Arham's family reportedly was a warm close-knit family who did most things "as a family". When he was asked how he managed to travel to places other than to the work experience placement, it soon became evident that he rarely travelled anywhere on his own: almost always with parents, friends, or siblings. Another aspect that became evident was that, though his family was deeply caring, that closeness came with expectations. His father was an engineer, and his mother a chemist. They wanted Arham to follow a similar profession, or at least something in the sciences, for that is where they considered future job security lay. They had been horrified when on one occasion Arham had suggested that he was attracted to becoming an actor.

To take a positive orientation, after asking about his family I asked him to tell me what he enjoyed doing. Aha! Reading, writing, poetry, taking part in the school plays, and enjoying listening to music. He had topped his class in English and languages. What one thing more than anything else did he simply *never* want to do, I ventured to ask? The answer came quickly: jigsaw puzzles, something that everyone else in his family was obsessed with. He just could not do them. His father was quick to interject, challenging him with not being interested. Further discussion revealed that he did not like watching films but loved radio. What was it about film and television that turned him off? He found it difficult to follow who was who as a film progressed, especially if there were costume changes.

Evidence was starting to suggest a possibility of *prosopagnosia*, a neurological disorder where individuals find it difficult to recognise distinguishing features of different *faces*. Noting he had become quite quiet as we talked, I felt it was time to again explore something positive before moving on. So I asked about his favourite novels, and discovered he had been writing a novel himself. The title was revealing: "The boy who got lost"! As he outlined the story it became clear that it reflected not just his experiences and understandings, but his fears of what could happen. It was the story of a boy who, from the description, experienced spatial disorientation, though he did not name it as such. In a traumatic event, his main character couldn't find his way home and, after accepting a ride from a stranger, was severely injured in a car accident. The character found himself in hospital suffering amnesia to the extent of not knowing who he was.

His story provided a segue into my use of a well-established low-threat interview technique: discussion in the third person. Here the answers to questions like "how do you think the boy *felt* at various stages?" were revealing. The process engaged him in what turned out to be an animated discussion. Arham clearly loved narrative, and on one level wanted to deepen his understanding of his book's character, so my explaining the psychology and neuropsychology of prosopagnosia and spatial disorientation meant that he was really engaged.

On another level he was also able to ask what would otherwise have been personal questions, questions that he may have been too shy or reserved to ask about himself, such as "did it mean the boy should be regarded as stupid?". As we talked, I was able to explain the nature of specific learning difficulties, and how they varied. He wanted to know about what sort of tests might help uncover them. This led naturally to suggesting he complete such a test, to understand his strengths and possible weaknesses.

In the last couple of decades there has been remarkable research into the structure of human cognitive abilities, resulting in a model that has become known as the Cattell-Horn-Carroll theory, CHC for short. The model is most comprehensively captured by the Woodcock Johnson assessment battery (WJ-IV).

Running Arham through the WJ-IV showed a gifted young man and, at a fine-grained level, clearly confirmed some interesting spatial difficulties.

Sharing this at a later session with his parents, together with Arham, we were able to set a pathway to realistic occupational expectations. It also led to exploring with him and his family some valuable ways of accommodating his difficulties. Some years later I found out that he had become a tireless and reportedly inspiring refugee support worker.

Learning difficulties mistaken for Youngest Child Syndrome

In contrast to the previous example, a young four-year-old was brought in by her quietly spoken parents: she seemed to them to be painfully shy. But they also suspected Brioni had a language difficulty: she would only speak in single words and only if no one else other than her parents or siblings were around. Her father was a radiographer and her mother a nurse. Brioni had two older siblings who were both doing very well at school.

They had been quite surprised that Brioni seemed quite happy to go to kindergarten, where she would play happily but always on her own, sometimes alongside others but she never spoke. The parents wanted to know if I could test her intelligence to see if she had some sort of language delay or disability.

What struck me about the parents as we talked was how quietly and matter-of-factly they spoke. Brioni in the meantime had taken up with some dolls from a box of toys kept in the consulting room, carefully moving things so that her back was to us.

As I turned to Brioni, she did not turn to me, seeming to ignore me while she continued to play. Her mother butted in, telling Brioni she should not be rude. Brioni pretended not to hear. I checked with her parents as to whether she understood, or whether her hearing was ok. They reported that at home she was able to follow any instructions, even when whispered to.

I sat down on the floor a little way from Brioni and picked up one of the other dolls and started to play with it. I started to talk to the doll I had picked up, calling her Emma. I had Emma speak back to myself putting on a voice I would expect from such a doll. Brioni continued to ignore me, not even looking around.

Her father broke in then, telling me that this was exactly what Brioni did at home if there were any strangers. This gave me an opportunity to take up a conversation with her father, aware that Brioni would be listening. I told him it was fine for her to do that if she felt she needed to. Then I went on to talk as from Emma, saying that not only was it ok, but that Emma knew exactly what Brioni must be feeling because Emma used to feel exactly the same way once. I then engaged Emma in further discussion. I explained to Emma that I could never *make* anyone talk, nor would I want to make anyone talk if they didn't really want to. I hoped that at the very least Brioni would turn around and look at me, but to no avail.

My conversation (as with Emma) continued, mainly about what Brioni was doing in her play, even surmising how she might be feeling. At the same time I engaged her mum and dad about their interests, what they enjoyed doing together as a family. While Brioni still did not turn around, her play slowed noticeably.

Quietly, Emma finally informed us all that it was time to finish and that she hoped Brioni would come back and play with the other dolls and tea set again next week. Emma then asked Brioni's parents if they thought Brioni might like to do that. With their positive answer we observed a surprising and unexpected nod from Brioni as she stood up, steadfastly not looking my way, walked over and took her mother's hand and headed for the door, with one quick wave to her doll.

I organised for the parents to set and leave a camera on a laptop in the family room rolling for a couple of hours one evening after the children came home. They then brought the laptop with them to watch with me. As always, initially the children were clearly seen playing up to the camera, the two older ones typically coming up and being exactly how children can be. As is usual, I suspect because there was no response, they then apparently became oblivious to the camera except for an occasional look across. Interestingly, Brioni kept her back to the camera, but as the other two relaxed and took no notice, Brioni was seen to move around, though not uttering a single word.

The video showed what looked like a typical family experiencing the mild 4 p.m. stresses: all a little tired after the day's activity and the children needing to tank some energy. What was most interesting, though, was to note how Brioni never spoke, yet the siblings and parents were always accommodating what she might want even before she pointed. At the meal table there was a lot of latitude given as she played with her food, with the father and mother both cajoling her quietly to eat up. Leaving a half-eaten meal after more than an hour at the table, she ran off happily when asked to go and have a bath her mother had run for her. We paused the video at various stages before and during the meal when someone was doing something for Brioni. I would ask the parents what they thought was going on. It was interesting to realise how neither saw any of Brioni's behaviours as anything that was voluntary, nor as her being in control. Rather, they had always considered she "could not help how she felt", so they simply needed to love and support her.

I reflected on Brioni's playing with Legos and her drawing. I then asked her mother to get Brioni to do some drawing at home, including a person, then the family, and then her favourite place, for them to bring to me.

> *"Draw-a-Person" or "Draw-a-Family" are techniques where the resulting figures can be scored to gain a rough idea of mental age.*

A picture of family, and the arrangement of the people in the family, can give clues as to how a child perceives their family, including their own place in it. The favourite place can often give a clue about happiness or fears, even potentially a sense of security or insecurity.

Be prepared to be surprised

Together we looked over the drawings. Her Draw-a-Family scored out as 12 months higher than age-appropriate. The family picture showed all standing together under a tree next to what looked like their home. There were clearly two parents, and between them and the two large children, a smaller child. Right over toward the edge of the paper was a drawing of a four-legged animal. It was easy to assume it was Brioni seeing herself as the centre of her family. But what to make of the dog right on the side? From the video and drawings, it looked to me as a normally functioning family, and it seemed that Brioni felt reasonably secure. I was forming one hypothesis: that Brioni had learned to be in control and looked after by playing helpless, and rarely speaking.

I suggested this to the parents, pointing out how, time and time again, Brioni's non-verbal pointing and delays at eating were rewarded by constant attention and help, from one of them. They were reluctant to accept this until I gave Brioni's behavioural patterns a name: "The Youngest Child Syndrome", whereupon an interesting and confirmative discussion ensued about position in families. This was only the parents' second session without their child, and up to this point we had clearly still been developing trust. However, with the discussion now on position in the family, joking and speculating about Eldest Child and Middle Child Syndromes, now we all were happily and personally engaged. I was able to suggest that I doubted Brioni had any cognitive (including language) disabilities and that, better than running some sort of testing, we should initially just look at appropriate behaviour modification strategies. This would need to focus on encouraging her to speak, with a determination to cease reinforcing Brioni's non-verbal requests. Time would then reveal any disability.

I had set up an expectation with Brioni to be returning to play with Emma. So, prior to their joint session, I rearranged the tea set and Emma in exactly the way Brioni had left them, having taken a photo before putting them away on the shelf. I had agreed on a discussion with the parents, purposefully crafted, to be overheard by Brioni. This included my saying that I considered Brioni a normal happy girl, capable of talking like everyone else, and that she would start talking once no one took any notice of her requests unless she asked properly. Throughout the session Brioni played happily yet was clearly resolute not to make any contact with me. It was as if I didn't exist. For me, it confirmed a very determined and aware, clever child, enjoying the Youngest Child Syndrome.

And so it proved to ring true. Over a couple of weeks, with a few phone calls, Brioni's parents consistently changed their patterns of behaviour reinforcement. Brioni had begun speaking in full sentences, though still tended to become silent whenever strangers were around. As an introvert, she might always remain shy, but in developing confidence this would not remain a problem for her.

Much of who we are is formed by the context in which we grow up. Understanding and working with children requires gaining a broad picture and working together with parents, family, and teachers. Unpicking the influences can be intriguing and surprising.

Jeffrey Young's Schema Therapy provides an outstanding evidence-based framework for understanding the influence of childhood experiences on development, including on attachment and beliefs that form into more complex schemas. We look more fully at that in the next chapter.

REFLECTIVE EXERCISES

Where do you see yourself in making any necessary assessment? Do you have the skills needed, or is it always important for you to know others to whom you can refer? I'm sure you will also have observed a cautionary note about running a battery of tests, simply to confirm someone else's opinion of the problem. The important additional caution here is not just to run those tests deemed appropriate, but to know how to properly interpret the results.

You will have observed how your necessary rapport with each of the clients may take different tacks. This is equally true for people of any age, and importantly will help avoid the potential for some clients to become tired or overwhelmed by assessments/tests that may never reveal the real issue. This is not to say, however, that testing will never be useful. In fact, some assessments can be very affirming, dispelling wrong beliefs about the self. Please recall some of the clients mentioned in previous chapters who so benefited from an assessment of their *real* abilities. More of this will be considered in our next chapter, under the section on Irrational Beliefs.

Chapter 16

Schemas that drive us

Problematic beliefs often underpin significant problems of adaptive adjustment. However, much of an individual's core belief system is mainly acquired through experiences in relational contexts, particularly during early childhood developmental stages which precede the development of any critical rationality. Working with maladaptive beliefs then needs to be both rational and experiential. A further exploration of beliefs that drive our behaviours and create internal tensions or belief sets are often conceptualised as schemas. These can be looked at through various perspectives, including different schools of psychology. Rational Emotive Behaviour Therapy (REBT) proposes a useful list of ten plus problematic irrational beliefs and proposes logical challenges to counter them. The general background to psychology and Schema Therapy is presented before looking at schemas. Some schemas not thoroughly understood are examined through case discussions which describe how to assist individuals who otherwise feel unable to move forward. Real reasons for seeking help also need to be uncovered, to identify thinking patterns that prevent well-being. Explanations of cultural schemas may form part of effective resolutions, particularly when cultural values are deemed absolute.

Is this the chapter I *must* write, perhaps *should*, or rather would *like* to write? Each of these statements leaves me feeling very differently about the writing, with not the least issue being the amount of stress I may experience! As mentioned in earlier chapters, self-talk can be so powerful – check examples in Chapters 1 and 5. However, we often don't recognise that these statements are driven by unconsciously held beliefs or set of beliefs that form what are called schemas. But more of these in greater detail a little later. Here we need to briefly consider some of the implications of holding troublesome or dysfunctional beliefs.

DOI: 10.4324/9781003474746-16

> *Dysfunctional beliefs that become problematic schemas have inevitably been taken on board uncritically, most often while young, when beliefs are simply and naively absorbed from the world around us.*

Recall young Tim, in Chapter 10, and his obsessions with being clean that resulted from an uncritical acceptance of an adult's pronouncement about his being a dirty little boy! Developmental research has found significant factors that contribute to the formation of ill-formed and debilitating beliefs. These include traumatic experiences, betrayed trust, problematic family attachment, physical and emotional abuse, unmet emotional needs, and even physical deprivation.

Must, should, and like to: control and responsibility

Bazhai was referred to me by a doctor "for assistance with chronic procrastination." She was in Australia to study medical science, hoping that this degree would enable her to qualify for getting into medicine.

When she was back home, Bazhai reported she had been a model student at the top of her class, fulfilling her parents' aspirations for her. Here in Australia, she now found far more enjoyment in going out and about socially with new friends. She needed to settle to study and did so for a short time. However, to her great surprise, gradually she found herself either impulsively doing other things, or just staring, overwhelmed by feelings she said she had never experienced before.

Checking things out found no indications of depression: she was sleeping well, eating well, socialising well. There was supporting evidence of her having good local social supports, including Singaporean friends who hoped to do the same course, and regular speaking with her parents. She had grown up speaking Singlish in Singapore as her first language, so no language problems there. She said she believed she had the abilities to pass all subjects she had taken on, and indeed had been looking forward with interest to studying. So why the procrastination? She sounded completely miffed about finding herself so easily preoccupied.

I asked her to think back to when she was procrastinating, feeling overwhelmed, or wanting to do anything else: what was the first thought that came to mind? She answered without hesitation: "I *must* get this done! I *have to* stop postponing! But the more I think that, the more I cannot stop procrastinating."

There was great passion in her using the word "must". I suspected that Bazhai would score as high, possibly problematically too high, on conscientiousness if given a personality indicator. So I probed a little about things she considered were important for her to do, even about recreational and enjoyable things, and her language in talking about them was peppered with the words "must" and "should" but few instances of "like to". I asked her how she went about organising each day, and that was when she said she felt most confused about procrastinating. She would make a list of all the things that she had to do, including setting a time when she must study after attending lectures and tutorials. Again, I noted how "must" was dominant, even in listing that she must catch up with certain friends, go to the gym, or call her parents.

There is a saying I like to use: the word "must" is like "mustard" – too *much* spoils the dish! But now was not yet the time for getting her to think about the conscientiousness that drove her. First I needed to explore her "must" in relation to her study, hopefully digging down to some potentially irrational beliefs using a process known as "chaining".[1] In this context, a counsellor keeps asking "why" in response to every answer, or alternatively, "what would having that [based on the answer] do for you?"

So, being sure to include the word "must", I asked Bazhai:

"Why do you think you must do this degree?"

Her answer was immediate: "To get into medicine."

"And why do you want to do medicine?"

"Because I want to help people, to make a difference."

Now I was at a branch in the chaining: I could ask why she wanted to help people, make a difference, but I suspected that there were other influences at play and it was time for a quiet probing low-level challenge:

"And why medicine? Aren't there other jobs to make a difference, help people?"

Bazhai paused, thinking. She was digging deeper. The answer came more quietly:

"Well, I have been told by everyone, you know, my teachers and . . . that I have the brains for it . . . and also my parents have impressed on me they think I must do medicine . . . and also [grin] I know they would be really proud."

Again, wanting to use the word "must" I continued to probe:

"So you *must* do medicine because it is the best use of your abilities for helping people, making a difference, and to make your family proud?"

"Yes . . . yes."

I allowed for a pause before asking:

"Do you think you will *enjoy* being a doctor? Nothing else you would rather do?"

There was a longer silence while she was obviously thinking, then her answer came slowly:

"I have never thought about how I would find being a doctor. I have never thought of doing anything else since my Year 8 home teacher said I should."

"So, do you think you will like being a doctor? Have you imagined the daily activities involved in the day-to-day work as a doctor? What if you find you really don't like it when you get there?" I probed.

The answer came slowly: "I don't really know."

"When you were younger, before Year 8, at primary school . . . what were you interested in . . . what did you like doing most . . . do you remember if you ever had any dreams of doing anything really interesting . . . when you left school?"

Bazhai sat reflecting before making a carefully considered answer. "I loved reading mystery and adventure stories, dancing, and acting in the school play and I thought people who were able to write stories were so lucky. I wrote some stories, and even a joke book! Never published anything, but friends who read them liked them, except mum and dad. They always pointed out I was good at maths and science, and as I went on, everyone told me I should do something really useful, like becoming a research scientist or doctor."

"Do you still ever write?" I was following a hunch.

"Why, yes, but I never share anything."

"And did you ever tell yourself that when you finish getting to be a doctor, you may pick up writing more ambitiously?"

"Um, yes, how did you guess?"

"So, you are headed towards doing medicine, not because you are attracted or know it is for you, but because you have been told that this is what you *must* aspire to, vaguely thinking that anything you really would *like to do*, must just wait?"

"Yes."

"What if we turn things around? How does this sound . . . and feel? 'Bazhai *must* write and possibly learn to act . . . go to acting school, and/or do an arts degree' . . . or 'Bazhai would *like to do* the day-to-day work of a doctor'."

I had turned "must" and "like to" around, and had also been careful *not* to say, "*become* a doctor", but "do the job". Bazhai was clearly a capable young person, so my assessment was that the challenges would be fully understood, and if so, we needed to bring any unconscious issues to the surface. I pondered what resistance, any hindrance from defence mechanisms with concomitant rationalisation, this might reveal. I allowed her time to reflect, and then her answer:

"I must be responsible."

I could have gone back to challenging her, even to argue about what being responsible looked like. But she had already indicated to me that she always tried to live up to other people's expectations of and for her. I needed to circumvent a common problem that I often observed: that so many people after a mid-life crisis finally pursue what they find intrinsically enjoyable and fulfilling, rather than continuing to put up with the stressful expectations and extrinsic drivers of their work commitments.[2] John Holland's Occupational Interests Personality inventory[3] was often useful at these mid-life times, but here was an international student having what I perceived was a pre-career crisis. Now to test the waters.

"Bazhai, I suspect you've had difficulty concentrating on lectures, not just getting down to study. It seems to me that even when you sit down for your scheduled study time, there is a part of you that maintains that you need to get on with your study, telling you that is being responsible.

"I am going to be very direct. I am not sure it is a problem of you not being responsible, but rather may be a personal requirement to live up to other people's and possibly even your own expectations, and potentially a matter of social standing. You couldn't tell me whether you were attracted to the actual day-to-day work of being a doctor.

"On the other hand, when you try to study, I suspect there is another part of you that deep down thinks this is *not* for you – and anytime that part of you has tried to raise that thought, you have consciously or unconsciously pushed it down."

Bazhai objected. So I listened to more about her thoughts about needing to be responsible, but then she went quiet. I gently continued. "I could be wrong, Bazhai, but reflect again with me. When you find yourself procrastinating, unable to concentrate, are you feeling just like you are tired, can't concentrate? Or are you sensing conflict, any conflict, deep within?"

Given time to reflect, she came to admit that, yes, she often felt conflicted, and it was as if she was hearing a fight within her.

Over the subsequent sessions we worked through her use of the terms "must", "should", and "like to", along with exploring conscientiousness and responsibility to herself, family, and friends. We touched on Real Self and Expected Self. We explored what it would be like in the long term for her to carry out the work involved in being a medical practitioner, including in various areas of specialisation. We explored her strong latent creative and artistic propensities, which emerged to the point where she recently had felt stifled when she could not be creative: socialising, having fun with friends, became her only compensation.

Being aware of your natural inclinations in the form of occupational interests can greatly contribute to thriving. Occupational interests are personality based, and may vary from or even be at odds with individual abilities and capabilities. Bazhai's experience illustrates how it is better to come to that understanding early in life. Conscientiousness should be about balancing one's own needs with the needs of others. If out of balance, aided by too much *must*ard, that stress can accumulate and compound with other life stressors.

Internal conflicts – faith and doubt

Ari came from a devout Greek Orthodox family. A caring paramedic, he was referred by his doctor for extreme anxiety at work around potentially making a mistake, and by not feeling appreciated or accepted by management. He made it clear that he had reluctantly agreed to seeing a psychologist since both his doctor and priest advised him to.

Why, he asked me, should he see a psychologist, and did his priest not help him? In faith he saw everything as in God's hand, and if he really believed God was in control, he should have no fear, and what people thought of him should not bother him. How could he be experiencing increasingly debilitating anxieties at work and now at home? His priest had confirmed that his beliefs about God were sound, but then he'd steadfastly insisted that the right psychologist could help him!

Ari went on without pause. He was even more worried now, just being here. Did he just lack faith? Surely this was a matter for a priest, not a psychologist. After all, he had been told that psychologists largely disregard people's beliefs and, even more, that psychology was anti-religious. In a debriefing after a traumatic work incident, one counsellor had told him that dealing with trauma had nothing to do with religion, as psychology didn't seem to be like theology or medicine in any way. Could I explain? He needed to understand, be reassured, before he could put any trust in me. Was I religious, and if so, what religion?

I pondered possible features of post-traumatic stress from his work experiences, so knew I would need to review any history of incidents. I also suspected at least two if not three of Rational Emotional Behaviour Therapy's (REBT) ten commonly held irrational beliefs might be his problem. But first, I needed to deal with his understanding of psychology and its many perspectives.

Brief background to psychology/philosophy/theology conflict

During a long discussion, with Ari asking many questions for clarification, I explained that Psychology has its roots in theorising: philosophy and theology. The first move from philosophy in claiming a move to a science was in medicine, when doctors were presented with severe mental problems. Sigmund Freud was recognised as a prime mover, with an approach now largely known as psychodynamic.[4] As the twentieth century rolled on, those wanting to move away from philosophising into what was regarded as much more empirical became known as behaviourists.

For radical behaviourists, the only real substance for a science is *empirically* verifiable: observable behaviour, antecedents, and consequences. Thinking (as thought processes) and beliefs were considered merely subjective and, as such, offered no useful substance or explanation for a *science* of psychology.

It did not make sense to Ari that beliefs were not important, as if they did not influence feelings such as anxiety. He asked: did psychology hold that his beliefs were irrelevant? Maybe psychology was right, and he was wrong, for despite his strong faith, he was increasingly unhappy. Did this mean that his faith was, well, maybe not strong enough, or perhaps misguided? Such doubts he did not like. I asked him to hold on, while I explained where psychology had gone.

I explained that during the second half of the twentieth century, behaviour therapists came back to *thinking*, when Cognitive Behaviour Therapy emerged. Cognition, I explained, is all about thinking *and* beliefs. To make the point that our reaction to everything we experience is determined by our beliefs, true or otherwise, I gave Ari an example I often use. If he saw two police officers outside a shopping centre, each with a revolver in their holster, how would he feel walking past them? He responded that he would feel really comfortable, since he often worked with police officers. Then I asked Ari how he might react differently if he'd just heard that a couple of murderers dressed in police uniforms were on the loose, looking to shoot up a shopping centre! We together explored the whole uncertainty created by our thoughts and beliefs that in turn affect our reactions.

I could then suggest that anxiety can come from a number of irrational beliefs that have been formed over time, though these might conflict with other quite rational and trustworthy beliefs. No matter how legitimate and true our religious faith might be, I assured him that we are capable of holding some irrational beliefs that give us trouble. I left him with some homework, to identify *the specific* implicit beliefs he held to be good and right, and which others were possibly doubtful, if not erroneous.

REBT – irrational beliefs

In the next session we went through his work history, cataloguing incidents that had been stressful and potentially traumatic. He came to understand how such incidents could result in troublesome beliefs. In the process we also went through REBT's ten irrational beliefs, some that in themselves may have some grounding, but when held as extremes, combined with self-talk using "must" and "should", can be destructive.

Control was a central issue for Ari, as is inevitably the case with most stress that continues post-trauma. We dealt with several traumatic events using Gestalt techniques. With Ari relaxed, he could visualise the incidents as if in his imagination, watching them on a screen, and with the remote controller in hand, he was able to control the film, even stop at times to walk in and talk to himself.

> *Can you reflect here on potential beliefs Ari held that may have been at best unhelpful and, at worst, quite troubling? Take time to review what you know of Ari.*

Hidden beliefs need to be exposed

The first belief for Ari that needed consideration was driven by his need to be competent and responsible in everything, but this unfortunately extended to his believing he should never make mistakes, especially not any serious ones. This in turn led to a belief that he never knew enough, and his feeling of inadequacy meant that he frequently needed to defer to others. Consequently, Ari refused to lead a team. As we explored these issues, we saw how an obsession with needing to be in control was clearly associated with previous experiences of trauma. Can you see the logical progression in the problem?

The second belief held at an *irrational* level was associated with his need to be liked and accepted by everyone, and most especially by people more senior to him or of importance, like his priest.

Working through these beliefs and needs, not only didactically but also with appropriate Gestalt-type dissociative activities, Ari subsequently gained a greater sense of control. It was encouraging to hear his wife report the changes she saw in him. Furthermore, Ari went on to encourage his elder son, a "chip off the old block", to also work through similar issues. Cognitive therapy, using the REBT framework, can be so effective and, in this case, Ari reported that it also helped him make more sense of his faith journey.

Schemas – beyond simple irrational beliefs

REBT and various forms of cognitive therapy more broadly developed over the last half-century, identifying stand-alone specific beliefs, irrational beliefs such as "I must do well and win the approval of others for my performances or else I am no good". Therapy involved straightforward disputation. More recently there has been a growing understanding of a greater complexity of beliefs as interrelated systems, with an appropriate way to deal with them beyond mere didactic challenges. Beliefs weave into what can be quite complex, interrelated bundles that Jeffrey Young, the originator of Schema Therapy, called schemas. Schemas are inevitably not held in any vacuum; they are typically and inextricably associated with need.

The case description above went beyond traditional CBT, being somewhat built on understandings from Young's Schema Therapy. Note just how Ari's *needs* were described almost interchangeably with beliefs and strong feelings. Unpicking the relationship between feelings, needs, and beliefs when brought into consciousness empowered Ari to make crucial decisions as to which beliefs were legitimate, and to clarify any that were destructive or contravened his values.

It is especially important to assist any client to nest amended beliefs and expectations within the values and beliefs held to be fundamental to their religious faith or personal convictions.

Background to Schema Therapy

The development of Schema Therapy has involved research linking schema formation to a combination of formative experiences and developmental factors. It also considered inborn personal characteristics and propensities: genes expressing themselves. This contrasted with the original development of behaviourism which sought to disassociate itself from psychodynamic schools of thinking and considered developmental understandings as largely an irrelevant distraction.

Jeffrey Young came from a practitioner background. This allowed him to adapt the commonly accepted *praxis*[5] by differentiating schemas. Young intrinsically knew that understanding how any problematic schemas had come to be developed was an important aspect that needed consideration in effecting change. With psychiatry's origins being psychodynamic,[6] many diagnostic conceptualisations, constructs, and terms in clinical practice still reflect psychodynamic origins. It is no surprise that as a practitioner, Young recognised the utility of understanding, particularly in terms of constructs that have their genesis in psychodynamic theories: personality, personality disorders, and attachment theory.

Ari illustrates an application of traditional CBT in the form of readily identifiable REBT irrational beliefs, beliefs that are held in the extreme. However, reading the case study, you can see that more elements were involved. Schema understandings were taken on board in relation to his beliefs system, conflicting beliefs associated with his religious commitment. But in Ari's case, there were no significant indications of problematic attachments past or present or of any personality disorders, so there appeared to be no need to look for problematic developmental experiences.

Remember: work deeply to identify the real reason for seeking help.

This moves us on to a more complex example: Bernice. As we went through the introductory pleasantries, I gained an initial impression of a well-dressed, well-spoken, and confident professional. On asking her what had brought her to see me, she looked a little uncertain as she handed me a GP's referral in an open envelope.

"Thank you for seeing Bernice, 48-year-old primary teacher, married, three children (all left home). Increasingly experiences problems of self-confidence, anxiety, particularly in social situations, with bouts of mild depression. She has seen three counsellors – expressed frustration. Currently seeking help from a homeopathist in lieu of conventional antidepressants. Not prepared to see a psychiatrist, but at the behest of her husband is willing to consult a psychologist."

On seeing me folding up the referral, before I could say anything, Bernice spoke, suggesting that "with all of that [I had just read]" she didn't want to waste my time as, really, no one could ever help her; no one could ever understand her. She was alone and different to anyone else she ever knew.

Through my mind ran several possibilities as to the subtext of this challenge: a reflection of despondency, doubt, depression, mistrust. Alternatively, was this visit simply compliance with another's wishes, while yet again verifying to everyone that she was beyond help? Or perhaps she really didn't want things to change? Such hypothesising too early can be a distraction. So first up, build some sort of rapport!

I suspected that in this case the rejected counsellors may well have done what we carers are all trained to do: practise genuine reflective listening! So, given her forthright manner and a suspicion that we might be looking at issues of control and potentially a personality disorder, it seemed more appropriate to run with her by agreeing with her: she might well be right, and quite probably I could not help or ever really understand her. However, nothing ventured, nothing gained, and since she was here now, I suggested we chat. It was clearly not an answer she expected, and a small wry smile showed as she nodded assent. I suspected she saw yet another opportunity for proving that she was uniquely beyond being helped. By this I surmised she was at least now feeling a little in control.

Asked to tell me about her family, she gave a very factual report. She had been married to a successful businessman for 27 years, had three sons, all doing well for themselves, while her parents lived 500 kilometres away, looking after her disabled brother since his motorcycle accident. Her husband's father had died when he was young, and his mother lived with her sister and occasional visits only were always with her husband.

What struck me about her report was its objectivity, focus on facts, and little if any emotion. When I asked about friends and what she did socially, there was a sudden show of emotion and a statement that, other than being with colleagues and at school-related meetings, she preferred to be on her own, knitting, reading, or watching TV.

Did she find it stressful being with others, I queried, to which she answered "no". She didn't find teaching or meetings stressful, just being with people socially, hating small talk. Encouraged to elaborate, she said that she had come to realise that no one really liked her, not even her family where she was unappreciated, and clearly not needed. Asked what evidence she had of this, she said that since her children had left home, neither her parents nor her mother-in-law ever visited; her children only ever came on a special day such as her birthday, and even then, without their partners. As for her husband, he was always working, even at night, at his computer or on the phone.

Again, this was all reported without any reference to feelings, so I nudged as to how she felt about how things were. Instead of answering as to how she felt, despite using the word "feel", she used it to report a cognitive belief that made her statement an explanation: "I feel things are just this way because, well, you see, I am different."

While the "why" question may be untimely early in a session, she had offered an explanation, so I probed further: how was she different, and in what way? Interestingly, Bernice's response was to challenge me, instead of explaining: how did I as a psychologist not see how she was different, and how that meant people simply did not like her? I needed to push towards feelings, so, noting that she perceived being unliked, I pondered whether she saw herself as unlikeable – even perhaps unlovable? With this she went quiet and looked down, clearly trying to contain emotions, and in an almost child-like vulnerable voice slowly answered: "Always! I have always been alone – always alone, always will be." Here I noted she was still reporting in facts. It was as near as I suspected she could come to verbalising anything emotional.

But it was her tone of voice that gave me some clues; my suspicion about seeing an age regression suggested some developmental trauma or unmet needs growing up. Another potential: to consider symptoms that suggested Autism Spectrum Disorder,[7] though the regression and repressed emotions appeared more likely to suggest a personality disorder.[8]

Schemas interpreted as coping modes

Much of the problem of boxing, or giving someone a label, was discussed earlier in Chapters 10 and 11.

> *The problem with a diagnosis of a personality disorder is that, by regarding the problem thus as a type of mental illness, it can be wrongly perceived as a life sentence, something to be endured and accommodated.*

A label only avoids entrapment if it is associated with an understanding of the drivers of a condition. Schema Therapy theory offers some handles that give leverage, particularly effective in relation to personality disorders. In terms of schemas, Bernice presented as operating in a vulnerable child mode, while her verbal avoidance of acknowledging anything emotional was best explained as a façade that served as a self-protecting mode for coping.

I was surprised when, at the end of the session, Bernice seemed to welcome my desire to speak with her husband, to know how he saw things. She articulated why she seemed pleased: because he needed someone to help him understand her, accept her as she is! Maybe this was a somewhat backhanded suggestion that she thought I understood her at least a little?

After gaining information from Bernice's husband and having further sessions with Bernice, it became clear that her attachment style, defensive modes, and associated schemas were indicative of a borderline personality disorder. The one repeating theme: no person had ever been able to convince her that she was lovable, and this included her husband and family, no matter what they did.

For many experiencing a personality disorder, there can be a resigned defeatism, not wanting to let go. Motivation can be difficult. In Bernice's case, though, she and her husband had acknowledged strong religion-based aspirational values, so over time these were able to provide some positive motivation for her to want to work on change. Care was needed to avoid any sense of guilt and any other sense of extrinsic control.

With necessary trust established, and working together with her husband, various techniques were utilised to both rationally and experientially tackle underlying schema(s). These included visualisations of past experiences as well as role-plays. A key to this was Bernice's capacity to stand outside herself and watch films of herself, recalling interactions with her parents and other significant adults in her early childhood years. Using her teacher training, it was interesting for her to realise that her coping within her professional role, as well as a mother to her children, meant expressing care in practical terms.

With Bernice's understanding of problem schemas and working them through therapeutically, a focus then importantly turned to the family dynamics, and family therapy proved very beneficial. Later one of her sons had explained: "I always kind of knew mum loved me because she shows it by what she does for you – but she never let me love her."

We hope another long example will not be too daunting, as we demonstrate how considering schemas can play such an important role in helping to clarify the issue. It's not an instance of the devil being in the detail, but rather that a greater insight and understanding is possible through the minutia!

Perhaps take a break here, before reading about schemas within the context of culture.

Culture as a set of schemas

Amara came with her grandmother Rosa. Amara explained that they were here because her grandmother thought they should come. After a brief pause, she added that her grandmother had very little English. So all questions and answers were translated for her grandmother, but, as I noted as the discussion progressed, with ever more shorter sentences to her grandmother.

Amara was about to turn 18 and was completing Year 12. She had been brought up by her grandparents after her parents had died in a car accident when she was three years old. The grandparents had wanted her to leave school after Year 10 and come home to work on their farm but had reluctantly agreed to let her finish secondary school. This had been possible after a long discussion with the school principal, a nun revered by her grandparents.

The new principal was a man, Mr O'Conner. He was now encouraging Amara to go on to university and her grandparents were angry. At this point Rosa, presumably having heard his name spoken, became quite agitated, saying "No good, no good, bad man".

Amara's grandparents had gone to see their parish priest. It was not for him to tell Amara what she should do, so he had suggested they take Amara with them to see me to help sort things out. They agreed only after he assured them I would agree with their beliefs – I suspected that had been a misinterpretation of his saying that I would either understand and/or respect them! Amara had now come in *without* her grandfather ("too busy on the farm"), and with some urgency as she needed to decide on accepting a scholarship.

It is quite draining when working with a translator, and even more so when one of the clients is the translator for the other. Even more problematic when another key person is absent. It was clear that Amara was very respectful of, if not deferring to, her grandmother, though I was unsure as to how much she may have been carefully filtering things. This led me to ask her to ask if Rosa might like to come in for a session with her husband and an independent translator, in order to hear their views. If so, then I would also see Amara on her own before seeing them together.

To my surprise Amara did not translate this to her grandmother but became upset. She assured me that her grandfather didn't need a translator, nor was he "the problem". Getting more upset, she went on to say it was her grandmother who wanted her to come onto the farm and to marry the 42-year-old bachelor and second cousin who owned the farm next door. Rosa now let out a deep sigh.

So, a clash of generational cultures. Psychologically speaking, cultures have been described as an inherently cognitive manifestation, as an expression of a set of beliefs and values formed together into cultural schemas. Cultures can also be understood as tribal. As such, what presented here can also be usefully thought of as a clash of religious, spiritual, and ethnic tribal schemas.

Going further in terms of schema theory, what of the unspoken needs and wants that were driving each? Maybe there were security needs for the grandparents in older age, while on the other hand, for a young person like Amara, perhaps there was a need for attachment and a sense of belonging in developing her identity?

Acknowledge cultural values collisions: no counsellor is value-free

This is to return to a theme we have stressed previously, and possibly most strongly in considering identity in Chapter 14. I have my own cultural schemas, with values strongly maintained around respect and individual rights. I live in an inherently individualistic rights-focused culture. This seems in tension with Rosa's collectivistic and protective compliance, honour-focused culture. It is a tension I sense Amara is experiencing. Clearly there is an attachment to her grandparents, and yet now a tension around unquestioningly accepting their *cultural* schemas. Does she need to capitulate, comply, or does she need to find herself, and if so, why and at what cost?

My values and beliefs inherently shape what I can provide as a service, and how. I needed to clarify these to Amara and Rosa, and so came my next request. I ask Amara to tell her grandmother that, like her priest, I cannot tell Amara what she must do. However, I ask her to explain that I am happy to see Amara and work on her making informed decisions for herself. If Rosa is happy for that, then we can progress, and I would also like to see her and her husband together, to fully appreciate their concerns.

Rosa leaves saying that she needs to talk with her husband. In the end Amara was able to come in for some sessions that allowed her to understand the tensions she was experiencing in terms of differences in cultural values driving schemas. The notion of tribalism was particularly useful for her. She recognised her grandparents' tribalism as being deeply rooted in their original home culture. She recognised the individualism of her local culture and was now able to make more informed rational choices while fully respecting her grandparents' beliefs. A key statement for her was that one can respect someone's beliefs, without having to agree with them.

The grandparents came in for two sessions. They expressed sorrow for Amara not taking on their treasured beliefs. They were able to say that they were primarily concerned for her happiness, but they also maintained that they knew best what would ensure a good life: honour. Amara did not feel able to take up a place at university for financial reasons. Family ties can be strong. She did convince her grandparents, however, to support her going to the local TAFE, where she completed a course in horticulture. She continued to live and work on her grandparents' farm, staying resolute however not to marry the boy next door.

REFLECTIVE EXERCISES

- Identify what schemas *you* may have developed that would impact any assistance you might want to give to people from different cultural backgrounds. Perhaps write them down.
- Then reflect on what beliefs are personally so important to maintain.
- Now consider which ones you may in fact be happy to challenge. Are they rationally based, emotionally based, or simply ones you thought of as a child, but need to fit with you the adult? Share your findings with someone you trust!

Notes

1 See Chapter 7 for another case example of chaining.
2 Remember other examples given like Sam, back in Chapter 2, and Tony, Chapter 12.
3 Holland's RIASEC Inventory: the interaction of personality and environment. Search on the internet for John Holland RIASEC, or Holland Codes; Wikipedia is excellent. There are numerous diagrams online, as well as self-help versions of Holland's Inventory.
4 Freud was interested in the dynamic relations between conscious and unconscious motivations.
5 Young demonstrates a *phronesis* by way of his schemas providing a basis to inform relevant practical action (*praxis*).
6 Wikipedia is an excellent place to start if interested in gaining a perspective on the nature and history of psychodynamic theory.
7 Autism Spectrum Disorder – for details, we recommend looking up Wikipedia.
8 Personality Disorders – as above, we recommend looking up Wikipedia.

Chapter 17

Interdisciplinary collaborations

With knowledge explosion has come an ever-increasing professional specialisation. The result of knowing more about less, the narrowing of focus, means that collaboration between specialisations and disciplines has never been more important. Effective collegial collaboration requires mutually respectful support, recognising expertise and accountability. Along with this comes both a sharing of duty of care and the need to understand boundaries. In this chapter we explore case exemplars that attempt to ensure ethical boundaries, while effectively engaging in mutual respect across helping professions.

Social worker

Rory and I enjoyed catching up over lunch from time to time. Consequently, these sessions had taken on a form of informal peer supervision that benefited us both.

Rory worked in a nearby country town with disenfranchised youth, some with various disabilities. His strengths: collegiate work, teamwork. Not only did his compassion drive him, but, being a high social extrovert and a realist he was personally energised when he simply could enjoy organising and doing practical things with people. He loved having fun, playing games, but also could turn his hand to helping "my supportie mates" as he called them, to sort out disorganised financial matters, or to challenge them to overcome bad habits or even addictions.

Not long into lunch one day, Rory became serious. There had been a complaint by a couple of other support workers, claiming that he had been breaching occupational health and safety regulations. It included the suggestion that he may have been inappropriate in some way or other, but he had been given no details of accusations. Rory was devastated when regional management insisted he take leave with pay while they investigated. I recalled he had previously shared how other support workers would often laugh and joke about him having such energy, such engagement with his clients.

DOI: 10.4324/9781003474746-17

Now, however, he was deliberately meeting up with me because the union lawyer had advised him to seek supportive counselling. It is a slippery slope for a discussion to move from peer discussion to counselling session. If he was wanting to move from colleague to client, there would be serious boundary issues. We needed to overtly clarify roles. In this case, as we talked it over, we agreed it meant formalising our time as peer supervision. To ensure ethical practice, appropriate transparency, and accountability, we agreed we would each keep formal notes and note these in our professional development logs.

In the longer term these notes and discussions proved to be invaluable in responding to employer and professional bodies' investigations. At the same time I was able to give Rory emotional support in a rough and challenging time.

Peer supervision as a matter of course for any one in helping professions is important, with increased benefits when this is across disciplines.

Welfare teacher

Armid was the student welfare teacher at the local secondary school. She was an experienced science teacher who had accepted the role somewhat reluctantly. She was appreciated by students in class because of her organisational skills, and her capacity to explain and clarify expectations. Six months into the new role, I had been asked by the principal to come to the school. Armid had asked for support from a school psychologist regarding a number of students with learning difficulties and others with unacceptable behaviour.

I was to learn about her inimitable practical and solution-focused way; she had made a three-column table, listing the students alongside "problem", and what she perceived was needed. This ranged from "intelligence test" through to "design of a behaviour modification program". Nowhere was there any term that might imply anything like counselling or social/emotional support.

Armid explained that the school budget was limited, and she wanted to get down to the business of providing psychological services to the students as efficiently as possible. She had set up a room where I could see each of the students listed one by one. The model Armid had assumed was a clinical one, and the only difference between a doctor's referral and this was that the sessions would take place at the school and not my consulting rooms. This left me with a dilemma. Should I just operate clinically and provide a report to the school, or was there the possibility of a school psychology role: support where I could work as a consultant, supporting Armid in her role as welfare teacher, and her assisting the students? How could I explain and negotiate what is perhaps a far more effective and efficient way of supporting students with difficulties?

Identify clinical roles versus those that are working alongside

The two models of operation have quite different implications in terms of responsibility: at base lies the question of asking who owns the problems that the students have? Working alongside teachers as opposed to a clinical model means that there is a sense of co-responsibility, and the opportunity to learn from each other. Over the years I have been greatly discouraged, if not frustrated, by the referral for clinical service of many students where there is an expectation that they are there for me to "fix" outside the context of the lived-in world.

This buck-passing is understandable: the demands on teachers in today's world are endless. Sidestepping the handing on, however, working *alongside* means that teachers have an opportunity for on-the-job professional development, giving them greater confidence by empowering them, through learning professional ways of understanding and working with student problems. It builds relationships of mutual support. But it takes time, a limited resource. When there is little time for engaging with teachers, extensive reports written after clinical assessments and therapy often seem simply to be filed and never really read, at least not by anyone other than the current teachers.

So, how to negotiate? I needed to understand and respect this welfare teacher's personality and worldview. She was direct, organising, and, I suspected, not inclined to unnecessary empathy. Negotiation was needed if I was not to simply fall in line with her expectations.

Though I was time-poor, I considered I needed to take time to develop a collegial relationship with the coordinator. So she agreed – initially somewhat reluctantly because of her own time pressures – that we set aside a session each week to discuss referred students. This soon developed into a wider discussion, including about handling students not referred. It also opened up opportunities for proactive preventative group work. In time, the coordinator reported feeling much more successful in her role, which I took to mean confident. The effect on resources was to reduce the number of referrals, and those referrals that were made were much more appropriate.

Cross-disciplinary teamwork brings many benefits. But specific roles need to be identified.

Chaplain

Alan had completed his psychology degree and taken up an appointment as a hospital chaplain. He approached me for supervision sessions to meet his 1,000 hours of professional supervised practice requirement for full registration as a psychologist.

There is a tension that emerges in terms of carrying out actual roles, and how they are perceived by others. A substantial part of his work needed to meet specific criteria of psychological practice, set out by the registration board to count as appropriate experience under supervision. Practising as a psychologist in Australia is only legally permitted as a registered health professional. While chaplains and counsellors may make use of psychology in understanding, they are not doing so as practising psychologists. This was clearly not the case for Alan as he was unambiguously counting at least part of his chaplaincy work as that of a psychologist.

The question then was: when was Alan practising as a psychologist, when as a chaplain, or when as both? Discussion had us draw a Venn diagram, two circles overlapping: one (chaplain) coloured blue and the other (psychologist) yellow, the overlap being green. We then drew up a table with three columns – blue, green, and yellow – and in each we listed all the activities he would expect to carry out in his work, including note taking, file keeping and professional development.

The question then arose as to the scope of my role as supervisor. Clearly, I was not his counsellor or mental health professional, though personal feedback and assessment should be an important aspect of supervision. After discussion, it became clear that he also needed a "spiritual" supervisor.

Finally, there was a question of how he would be perceived by patients and staff. Anyone he worked with as a psychologist would need to give their consent, fully informed. How could this be done simply? Firstly, both his employer (a church-funded agency) and the hospitals where he would be working needed to be fully informed of blue, yellow, and green activities, and to give considered consent to him carrying out both roles. Secondly, a name tag for him was devised clearly indicating "Chaplain and Psychologist". Thirdly, we composed a simple handout which he could make available to anyone asking for more detail. Jokingly he suggested that maybe he needed three differently coloured hats he could wear as appropriate!

In the ensuing supervisions there was a realisation that the boundaries between the three areas were much fuzzier than they appeared initially. There was an argument that in all his work he was a psychologist, bound by well-defined professional ethics (set out by the registration board), as well as the requirement of practice being evidence-based. It brought up many interesting discussions as to his sharing the Christian gospel, and as to whether praying with a patient or stressed staff member was considered in any way appropriate, indeed, as therapy – or not!

Perhaps a good time to *reflect*: how would you answer those various issues raised?

Clergy person

Clarissa, a clergy person, came to see me asking for supervision. She was new to a difficult and small parish. There were several strong and forceful long-term members, each with projects over which they exercised an authoritarian control. Then there were a number of non-engaged parishioners who came to worship services, many only sporadically. Occasionally these individuals would support one or other project, but Clarissa had seen many withdraw when all they were permitted to do was follow instructions. Moreover, Clarissa recently had been told to keep herself to her role as a clergy person. She assumed that meant she was expected to keep out of any of the church projects considered the domain of males, including anything like building maintenance!

Asking for clarification as to what she wanted from a psychologist, she indicated that she had a spiritual director/supervisor that she perceived as supporting her role as a pastor/minister, but she wanted psychological advice on dealing with a rigid church culture. She also expressed the need to learn ways of personally being assertive *in a constructive way*, to deal effectively with any conflicts that might arise.

Clarissa had come asking for supervision. She already had supervision relevant to her profession, so it seemed to me that rather than asking for counselling or therapy, she was in fact asking for interdisciplinary support: organisational psychology leveraging social psychology. Was supervision the appropriate term to capture the role, or more appropriately consultancy? We discussed what each of the roles might involve, and that clarification was significant in setting our directions, including specified goals.

> *Working effectively in interdisciplinary teams requires explicit clarification of roles and expectations.*

Setting goals

The consultancy provided reading material, discussion, and role plays, almost a bespoke course. In this case the consultancy was limited to working specifically with Clarissa, and included feedback following a personality indicator, ways of thinking and coping, and looking at her Achilles' heel. This meant that in dealing with any church culture problems, I had to rely on Clarissa's perceptions and understandings and be reasonably confident that these were sufficiently accurate.

A more ideal situation would have involved working with the congregation, or at the very least, the church leadership team/elders; however, that was unlikely to be acceptable. Clarissa reported a seemingly large block of entrenched congregants who no doubt were well intentioned, but certainly resisted change. A more systems-centred approach would have been to set up a respectful review by all within the parish before goal setting could be effective.

Importantly, Clarissa reported finding it particularly helpful to come to understand the concept of problem ownership: to reconsider the situation in terms of the congregants not seeing that there was a problem, unless she were to push for change! On the other hand, Clarissa had a problem (or problems) in what she perceived as her responsibilities, given a problematic and rigid church culture that excluded many from any real sense of empowered involvement and belonging. Simply put, she finally grasped that her church had developed an authoritarian culture, so that certain strategies had to be developed to achieve desired change.

Among other things, systems theory offered a mapping of relationships and forces to maintain the status quo. As the consultancy progressed, Clarissa learned that even the softest nudge towards change needed strategic tact and patience, and a load of support and frequent debriefing for herself. Unrealistic expectations would only serve to cause frustration, with a potential for burn-out. Much of this work was also supported by her spiritual director.

A small parish can be intense. Despite outside support, being the only clergy person, Clarissa expressed she was lonely. Over three years she developed some useful conflict management skills, patience, as well as the ability to set realistic expectations, but the opportunity to join a team ministry elsewhere proved too attractive. In her final meeting she told me that, much as she loved the people, tongue in cheek, she thought she had spent enough time in the purgatory of their difficult culture.

I could not help asking her what she meant by loving the people (with an implied "why, if you love people, would you leave?") and her answer was simple: "I care for their wellbeing, but I am frustrated in not being able to do more in helping them . . . in the way they relate to others, in the way they help others and support each other. If I stay there much longer, I fear I may wind up having to ask for forgiveness for not loving them as I am commanded."

REFLECTIVE EXERCISES

Reflect here about how you see your own role connecting with others who either supervise or do the hands-on caring. It may also be helpful to reflect again on the well-known serenity prayer attributed to Reinhold Niebuhr (see Chapter 4).

Chapter 18

Caring for the carer

Since this book has been written with a wonderful variety of helpers in mind, we believe the focus of our final narrative needs to reflect with you as you variously support a vast pool of needy folk. All of us in caring for others also have our own specific needs, and our hope is that you personally may benefit from reflectively thinking through some of these issues. Here we explore some of what we see as core issues that carers commonly experience.

This chapter may also provide helpful insights relevant to those you support who are in fact doing the demanding heavy hands-on caring of others.

Potential unmet carer needs

Carers are people who are mostly givers rather than takers.[1] Perhaps you are more aware of the complicated stressors that carers as givers experience because you know first-hand what that involves.

> *Jot down some points you believe are some of the most difficult aspects of caring for others.*
> *As a carer, evaluate how well you think you cope.*

For you, stress issues may be more about feeling emotionally stretched, or coping with hearing the details of others' pain which can be very draining. The challenge of taking in what is shared while also trying to "keep your head above water", is quite challenging.

Maybe you find yourself thinking about some of the common carer problems that are expressed in awkwardness, not knowing how to handle people who are different, lacking understanding about individual differences. We hope you may have gained some insights suggested by our earlier chapter on personality.
We have found that people can spend a lifetime frustrated by the very people they have lived with for so long but never understood!

DOI: 10.4324/9781003474746-18

Perhaps other carer problems demonstrate very deep unmet personal needs. Often unexpressed, such personal needs can frequently somewhat mistakenly seem to be selfish, even unreasonable. You may have observed that caring without adequate support or encouragement is a common issue that many struggle with. You may have also observed difficulties that some carers experience when there is a clash of values between them and the one being cared for. And what about the very real concerns for the "patient" who, though showing signs of dementia, still expects to be treated as ably independent?

Let's imagine that your role, however, is as an outsider, trying to equip a carer who needs to feel more able to cope. The focus then is on how *your* understanding of their needs can be effectively translated, mirrored back to them, and by so doing can leave you feeling somewhat uplifted too!

Habits from the past

We recall Vera, briefly referred to in Chapter 14, who sought support, trying to manage caring for an elderly parent, while also trying to keep up the ordinary demands of her immediate family. She was used to being busy, she said, but the worst part now for her was trying to figure out what were the *necessary* tasks as compared with the tyranny of the *urgent* ones.[2] Taking in her details included not just absorbing the numbers (four children and a husband) but asking questions to know what she and her husband as parents had learnt as children about the value of sharing and caring, and how that now operated within their present family.

As a child, Vera had been expected to work hard on the farm while she lived at home. Now living in town, she valued seeing her children being happy kids, not expected to contribute to any of the menial regular tasks thought to be hers. Her husband Joe was often away truck driving, so Vera's role as the mother meant she was always overtaxed for time and energy. Since her widowed mother had been unable to live alone, she had been moved into their only spare room. Her mother virtually never left her bedroom, being quite restricted by a number of physical disabilities.

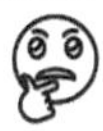 What other questions do you have that need answers, so that you might best support Vera? Can you imagine any personal, more emotional needs that might also unwittingly be creating additional stress for her?

Remember: she has come to you because she expects to gain further insights than those she has already thought about on her own.

The carer's emotional needs

Feeling the physical effects were quite easily alluded to, as Vera acknowledged there were not enough hours in the day to get everything done – "feeling worn out" was her best description. But other feelings needed to be explored and questions asked: how easy was it for her to do things for her mother? Was her mother ever grateful, and patient, for example, if Vera was not immediately responsive? And when Vera was called away, did her children behave well, willing to help Gran? I also asked about her own freedom to call in help, even if Gran did not like her privacy being invaded.

You see, what needed to be explored were the elements of feeling overwhelmed that might be somewhat relieved simply by involving other people. This meant engaging Vera in self-reflection: what was her rationale for never expecting the older children (now nine and 12) to help with at least some of the chores? Her answer revealed some strong feelings of resentment, her having to do everything on her own, but when these were further scrutinised, Vera admitted it was easier and quicker to do the chores herself. That in itself raised some concern about how insistent she always was about the way things should be done. Such reflection also allowed Vera to recognise how she had neglected the teaching role she could have utilised, and from which she had benefited much as a child. A sense of responsibility which had become second nature to her, but which she now saw was missing within the family dynamics.

Love for her children was not in question. She admitted she had formed an unhelpful *Ideal* self-belief, that she *should* be able to do all the things she used to do for them, but now expressed feeling guilty, particularly about dividing her attentions away from them to her mother. She admitted she had begun to feel real resentment there too: caring for her mother, having to do everything for the children, and eventually dared express her childish resentment about washing her husband's clothes! Some feelings of guilt needed to be exposed as false guilt. Along with this was my affirming that her best intentions could never guarantee she would be able to get everything done as she would have liked to.

Exploring guilt, grief, and resentment

Speaking openly with the children to engage them in caring for her, their own loving mother, was not as difficult as she'd thought: new behaviours now expected of them became growth opportunities for them. They now understood how their mother felt, so they newly explored with her how they could help. Vera also appreciated encouragement to consider ways of enlisting outside help for her own mother: inviting others to visit and read with her, to alleviate some of the stress of being so alone; considering meals on wheels; asking for community assistance with showering, etc. Though initially she believed it wrong to make her mother accept outside help, she could see the alternative as being potentially far worse, should she need to be moved into institutional care.

You may also understand how Vera's grief had not been identified until she was given the opportunity to explore her own less immediately obvious feelings. She clearly needed an outsider perspective on her own needs, as well as those seen in her failing mother. In fact, Vera's deep grief was finally admitted to, and with some emotion. Her mother had always been so capable, but now she almost had to be treated like a child. Vera felt conflicted by this, as if she had become mother to her own mother, now the child. She had to express sadness and loss over this . . . before a new reality was finally allowed in. She could not stop the ageing process, and for her loving care to continue, she needed to make choices about what changes were required. Some of these were impossible without adaptations, and others being involved.

Personal reassurance supports self-determination

Affirmation about all that Vera had been doing was an important part of our interactions, with personal encouragement and understanding coming from the less emotionally involved third party. This helped confirm her decision to take action, to give herself permission to make those changes, and now, without fear of self-condemnation. She could see how she had been stuck with certain misbeliefs that had previously prevented her from clearly making priorities. She learnt again the power of accepting that what needs to occur might not always be appreciated by all impacted by such decisions.

Any changes that an individual wishes to make necessitate a preparedness to be adaptable. Sometimes this revolves around the circumstances that are ever evolving, often unpredictably, so someone in a carer's role also needs to be aware and willing to adapt or sometimes, even to withdraw. However, an awareness of what changes the other is experiencing is also important, to still be able to encourage treasured independence as long as possible. This needs to run in tandem with caring for your own needs, which often is quite challenging.

> *Ensure that every carer maintains an appropriate level of self-care, regardless of the pressures they are experiencing.*

As earlier seen by cases given in Chapter 10, this can be extremely difficult when caring is no longer possible because of another's drug dependency.

Complications of drug dependency

An elderly couple comes to mind: William and his wife Beth, both in their early 80s. They were uncomfortable asking a stranger for help, but a friend had said that psychologists were good listeners! Beth needed reassurance that it was "alright to come to talk about their son". They were assured that I was happy to have them share about him, but that I could really only seek to offer realistic help to *them*, not to their adult son. It was soon apparent that the focus indeed needed to be about themselves. Yes, they did believe their son Trevor had a serious drug habit, but they couldn't seem to get him to take responsibility for that addiction. For years they had supplemented his income, so that he was able to live independently, as he wished to be "closer to the city". They described his accommodation as distressing for them to even visit, given his disinterest in keeping it clean, on top of his being less than welcoming to his generous and caring parents. But then, being benefactors implies doing well by helping someone, doesn't it? So it was important to ask in what way their financial help was really helping Trevor.

This was where some of their personal issues became more obvious. Beth had long been emotionally committed to providing whatever Trevor said he needed. But William would have seriously prevented this much earlier on, except that Beth insisted they must continue to love their son. "He has no one, we have each other!" was her defence. It was important to ask them individually what their respective understanding of care meant, so that in the safety of a third person with a more objective perspective, they could disagree with each other. My role was to listen as they each explored their understanding of love, and to steer them to honestly consider how well that had really worked for Trevor.

When caring becomes too tough

Can you grasp the picture? Both loved their son, but their individual abilities, inclinations, values, and beliefs had not prevented Trevor becoming less and less able to be responsible for his own choices. And there was the additional reality, expressed by William, in his fears for what would happen to Trevor when they could no longer keep up their financial support. They also worried what he'd do after they died. They then expressed a desire that Trevor should see a psychologist, to make sure he was doing ok. The question of his acceptance of there being a problem was in their view unanswerable. They were hoping that he would answer that honestly himself.

It was agreed that Trevor be asked to attend, to allow someone else to assess if he were managing. This was on condition that he willingly made an appointment, and with the full knowledge that his parents had been before him.

Before the parents left, some valuable time was spent in understanding how well they were looking after themselves, and what realistically they hoped for their son. This also meant they needed to become aware of the potential that their son would not even admit to having any problem. This fact was gently driven home, leaving them aware they still had a decision before them about their role in

Trevor's future. They were left with the task of asking him, for their sake, to make an appointment within the next month. They agreed they would attend again after that time, regardless of whether Trevor had or had not agreed to their request.

It was some surprise to me that he did arrive for an appointment. And from all that he shared, there was no willingness on his part to believe he had a drug dependency; he considered his drug taking to be well under control. There were some strong indications of schizoid ideas, with his tendency to live in a world of self-belief that was irreconcilable with other contradictory statements about what he was achieving. There was not enough information given to know whether these expansive ideas were drug-related or otherwise. Trevor described his relationship with his parents as good, though he reported being too busy to know much about how they were. He thought they'd always worried about him, but there was no need. And certainly, he was quite sure he needed no help; he was happy where he was living and didn't need any interference from them or anyone else.

This elderly couple made their next appointment, with a hope expressed by Beth that their son might have agreed to ongoing help. I'm sure her wishful thinking had resulted in William frequently trying, over the weeks prior, to convince Beth it was very unlikely that Trevor would admit a need for help. Trevor had given me permission to tell them all about his visit, indicating he had no worries, and they had no reason to worry about him!

Did they need to know the truth? To hear my understanding of where Trevor was at? *Their* needs, while considering themselves to be Trevor's carers, were still my priority. The contradictions I had observed, both in his expressed ideas, his body language, and the stories about what he was supposedly creating, were sadly shared with them, and even more distressingly received. They themselves knew the truth, but they needed to hear it from an objective perspective, and to express their distress. Quite sad to be part of. Silence was needed, before William asked the inevitable: "what then should we be doing?"

Can you see what even the *asking* of such a question meant to them? They had come to a dead end. But what could be said to make things easier for them to accept – was there *anything*? Even my having shared the little I had gained of my perceptions of Trevor's life of lies and self-delusions was heavy enough for them to hear. But they finally accepted what they had long suspected: they could not continue to believe his strange denial of the truth. His drug habit had taken their son from them, and their admirable attempts to help him were currently of no benefit.

They had few relatives who could support them, and fewer friends on whom they wished to depend. Their son had been their life, and for so long. William had decided he would let Trevor know they could no longer afford to financially support him. This prompted a caution, that William did this in a safe way, with a support person present. They also recognised that they could not ever let him move back home, to live with them. Other fears were grudgingly finally admitted to, including their genuine concern that he did not care about *their* future, so they both understood they had to take care of themselves.

In this way, my caring for them needed to be relinquished to others, who were appropriately found within the social network for people at risk. They agreed for me to contact and share their story with a well-known social worker. In allowing that visit to them, they still hoped others might also visit their son, should he become more willing. It was important to encourage them to follow through this alternative place of support, with an awareness that Trevor might yet return with demands they really could not provide.

Another example of an elderly carer

The same heaviness was observed in a lady, then in her mid-70s, who presented as tired and anxious. But her reasons for attending were not selfish concerns but rather for her only daughter, now in her mid-30s and very dependent on her parents. As a mother, Patrice shared how she had wonderfully cared for this child: Narelle suffered from a genetic disorder, with facial characteristics of a person with Down Syndrome, but she was believed only as having a mild to moderate intellectual disability. Narelle loved cooking, and even demonstrated an independence about recipe reading, decision making about cleanliness habits, and an ability to learn if clear instructions were given.

As has been demonstrated with so many of the cases described throughout this casebook, the ostensible story of Patrice's distress was not the total picture. Patrice worried what she could do to prepare her daughter for a time when she would not be able to be her carer. Gentle questioning revealed a husband, Neil, who had tried to keep his daughter out of the public eye – ashamed of her appearance and disabilities. The real issue had come to light: why the daughter had not been exposed to greater opportunities for developing independence!

It took two sessions for this mother to gradually see what was important to consider for her daughter's sake, not for her own. This involved her having to face her husband's annoyance and his possible anger at her ostensibly choosing to go against him. During these sessions, she was then encouraged to deploy her self-confidence more specifically, learning appropriate ways to deal with Neil's perspectives, *before* sharing a new way ahead for Narelle. Again, this necessitated teaching the difference between simply maintaining a submissive agreement with Neil or being prepared to be assertive on her daughter's behalf.

If you need to refresh your understanding, refer back to Chapters 2 and 4, and the appropriate use of saying what you need to say without aggression, and without the need to simply and passively back down.

Patrice had long lived with the consequences of this latter choice, and she began to understand the impact on both her authoritarian husband Neil, but also more on Narelle. Post-primary school had virtually seen her withdrawn from social contacts – apart from some of her mother's friends who occasionally visited. Narelle lived very much in fear of her father and had developed an unhealthy suspicion of people in general.

As an aside here, one should note that the longer a status quo has been accepted, the more difficult it is for the perpetrator of that stance (as in Neil's dominance over his wife and daughter) to be considered worthy of change. He could be excused for assuming in this case that he was right, simply because Patrice had gone along with his demands. Standing up to him took courage. But her love won through, so that like many in that situation, Neil finally gave up, wiped his hands of his daughter, and allowed Patrice to have her own way, so long as nothing was demanded of him. Perhaps her determination ultimately made him see the end of what holding his attitude would mean for Narelle. Maybe his own age, well into his 80s, and associated vulnerability, enabled him to accept the inevitability of important changes.

Not only was my role with Patrice to encourage her to voice her daughter's unmet needs, but to enlist the help of her few friends in finding out about alternative places of "work" for someone with special needs. This then meant that Patrice needed to talk more openly with Narelle about a way ahead, so that her initial fears about "making it alone" could be dismissed. A growing programme of deliberately exposing Narelle to public transport, initially always with her mother, was then followed up by choices of selected places to go, all which would eventually mean more independence. The challenges were many, but Patrice was still young and able enough to take these on board while she had strength and determination.

This case was quite an astonishing one to me, as it reflected a bygone age I had thought to be well past. But it again demonstrates the core issue: to those important questions, interpretable answers enable any individual to bring about crucial personal changes, so long as they grasp hold of "where there is a will, there is a way". We may not be asked or be able to literally hold that person's hand through that journey. But we may be asked to help them envisage the possibilities, and grant them personal insights, some of which may have been lost along the way. In turn, such understandings can strengthen their resolve to take up the challenges associated with continuing to care for others.

IN CONCLUSION – A FINAL REFLECTION

You may have frequently heard people offering concern and even pity for someone who has suffered a tragic injury, or a serious illness that has left them very debilitated. But hopefully you also registered that there is often a commensurate *neglect* to express any cognisance about what the *carer* themselves may or will be experiencing. Sometimes the carer's quality of life is severely diminished, with no relief apparent on the horizon. This is particularly likely if they carry that responsibility alone.

Several examples come to my mind. Think of young parents, burdened by a child with a terminal illness, or limited life expectancy through a disability. Sometimes this heaviness has been known about from infancy, or it may be a newly known truth that is so hard to believe and accept. This grief is even more tragic when a sole parent has to carry this alone.

If these examples are part of your personal experience, regular times to reflect with a trusted confidante about what you are really feeling is so important. Another's healthy perspective can often be an open window that allows a distant or alternative horizon to become more visible, more worth trying. But, if you are supporting such a person, remember again that ownership of *their* problem is not yours to carry; your role is to be supportive, encouraging, and sensitively reassuring of your love and concern for them.

This book is a casebook about caring for others: our hope is that you have been encouraged by reading it. In the face of a mountain of human problems, it can be a joy to offer a hand that makes a difference, if only for some. That giving comes at a cost, however, and always needs to be balanced against self-care, for personal well-being. As encouraged throughout the book, making a habit of personal reflection is essential, if we are to find and maintain a healthy balance between giving and taking, between the needs of those we serve and our own.

At this moment of writing, we watched the newly released Australian film, *The Way, My Way*, based on the bestselling book of the same name. It is an enjoyable, truthful, and thought-provoking reporting of Bill Bennett's personal pilgrim walk through Spain along the Camino de Santiago. It is a beautiful reminder that life is a journey of many layers, not the least being the need to be supporting one another.

As we journey on, may we remember: "there is a time and a season for everything."[3]

Notes

1 *Give and Take* (2013), a book by Adam Grant provides further reading that looks at "Why helping others drives our success", and is a valuable insight into an additional way of understanding the people in team work who are not easily accepted or understood.

2 See Charles E Hummel's 1967 booklet, *Tyranny of the Urgent.*

3 Ecclesiastes 3: reflected on by The Seekers.

Index

Kolibri 360 GmbH
Ferdinand-Jühlke-Straße 7
99095 Erfurt, Deutschland
produktsicherheit@kolibri360.de